Child Abuse and Neglect

Edited by Michael Fitzgerald

Published in London, United Kingdom

Child Abuse and Neglect
http://dx.doi.org/10.5772/intechopen.98096
Edited by Michael Fitzgerald

Contributors
Sílvia Fraga, Mariana Amorim, Sara Soares, Robyn May White, Juan Bornman, Ensa Johnson, Sunha Kim, Amanda B. Nickerson, Tia E. Kim, Rosalba Rombaldoni, Vittoria Ardino, Elena Acquarini, Keva Bethell, David Allen

First published in London, United Kingdom, 2022 by IntechOpen
IntechOpen is the global imprint of INTECHOPEN LIMITED, registered in England and Wales, registration number: 11086078, 5 Princes Gate Court, London, SW7 2QJ, United Kingdom

British Library Cataloguing-in-Publication Data
A catalogue record for this book is available from the British Library

Additional hard and PDF copies can be obtained from orders@intechopen.com

Child Abuse and Neglect
Edited by Michael Fitzgerald
p. cm.
Print ISBN 978-1-80355-510-2
Online ISBN 978-1-80355-511-9
eBook (PDF) ISBN 978-1-80355-512-6

Meet the editor

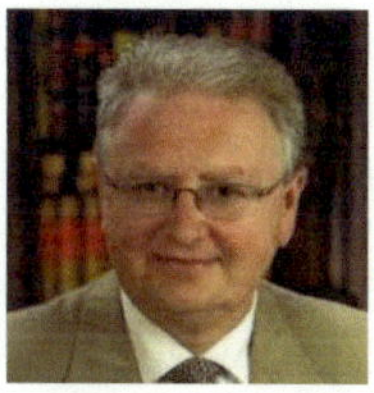

Professor Michael Fitzgerald was the first Professor of Child and Adolescent Psychiatry in Ireland specialising in autism spectrum disorders (ASDs). He has diagnosed more than 5000 persons with ASDs. He has written many peer-reviewed publications and authored, co-authored, and co-edited thirty-four books, some of which have been translated into Japanese, Dutch, and Polish. Professor Simon Baron-Cohen, world-renowned expert in clinical psychology and professor of developmental psychopathology at the University of Cambridge, described one of Professor Fitzgerald's books on autism as, 'the best book on autism' and described him as an 'exceptional scholar'. Professor Fitzgerald has lectured extensively throughout the world, including at the Royal Society/British Academy and the British Library in London. He was the overall winner of the Excellence in Psychiatry Award in 2017 and was nominated as one of the top four psychiatrists by Hospital Professional News Ireland. Professor Fitzgerald recently retired to spend more time in Brussels and continues to write on autism.

Contents

Preface

Child abuse and neglect are one of the greatest challenges facing psychiatric, psychological, social, and health services. Its prevalence is increasing due to numerous factors, including migration, war, poverty, and even climate change. All members of the psychiatric, psychological, social, and medical professions need to be attuned to it, not only in identifying it but also in intervening for persons who have been or are being abused. It presents a massive public health challenge. This book is timely and is meeting the challenge of these major adverse events on child development, the effects of which can last a lifetime.

Violence has a major impact on child development.

In Chapter 1, Bethell and Allen show how group therapy helped in the resocialization of a traumatized group in Barbados. Many of the individuals had adverse childhood experiences and many also had post-traumatic stress disorder. This chapter shows that resocialization through group therapy has considerable potential as an intervention in marginalized groups.

In Chapter 2, Acquarini et al. examine developmental trauma through the lens of public health and discuss its implications for health and social care as well as society as a whole. They emphasize a trauma-focused public health approach. They also elaborate on a new disorder called developmental trauma disorder.

In Chapter 3, Fraga et al. distinguish between repetitive violence over time and isolated incidents of violence. They take different contexts into account, including home and school. Violence can have long-term diverse effects on personality and may be associated with psychiatric disorders. Resilience is key and one must be mindful of it.

In Chapter 4, Kim et al. focus on improving the teaching of child sexual abuse (CSA) knowledge with training, which should have the effect of improving the identification of persons suffering from CSA. It has been estimated that as many as 28% of youths 14–17 years old are exposed to CSA in the United States. The authors analyze their findings using a latent mediated structural equation modeling approach. The interventions were successful in improving the level of knowledge of teachers who had initially lacked CSA knowledge.

In Chapter 5, in a legal scoping exercise, Bornman et al. describe court accommodations for children with disabilities via a literature review. This is of critical importance if justice is to be had. Children with communication disorders are particularly at risk of child abuse and neglect.

Michael Fitzgerald
Professor,
Trinity College,
Dublin, Ireland

Chapter 1

Resocialization through the Family Project in the Bahamas: Using Group Therapy to Heal Adverse Childhood Experiences

Keva Bethell and David Allen

Abstract

Background: The Bahamas has undergone a severe social fragmentation process due to the crack cocaine epidemic of the 1980s. Marginalized persons were offered free group therapy through The Family: People Helping People Project. Methods: We hypothesized that many of our participants were traumatized as children, therefore causing them to experience various psychological and physiological challenges as adults. The Allen Resocialization Scale can measure the resocialization of traumatized participants. Results: The results indicate that 98% of participants who were traumatized scored 'excellent', 'good' or 'average' on the Allen Resocialization Scale. Conclusions: Without The Family, these participants may have been 'poorly' re-socialized, wreaking havoc in the society. Therefore, the results suggest that Family support groups can be a protective factor against trauma experienced in childhood.

Keywords: adverse childhood experiences, post-traumatic stress disorder, family, resocialization, group therapy

1. Introduction

The Bahamas is a small island nation situated between Florida and Cuba. Originally an English Colony, it became independent in 1973 and had a population of about 400,000, most of which is of African descent. The Bahamas is a religion-centric country based on Judeo-Christian principles. Unfortunately, the country-wide crack cocaine epidemic of the 1980s produced severe family and community disintegration [1, 2], which, combined with the international economic downturn of 2008, led to high youth unemployment and the development of violent gangs. In response to this, The Family: People Helping People Project, a resocialization intervention, was initiated in 2008 [3, 4]. The program provides free group therapy to 23 marginalized communities, including the prison, juvenile offenders, and an orphanage. The Family is a group process model, representing a therapeutic replica of the home-based family, allowing members to confront their issues in a safe and non-judgmental environment led by a trained facilitator. The Family provides support and advocacy for its members, which in turn gives persons an avenue to discover themselves and grow as individuals [5]. More importantly, The Family encourages the expression of taboo emotions, such as early childhood trauma. Study findings repeatedly reveal a graded dose-response relationship between adverse childhood experiences and negative health and well-being outcomes across the life course [6, 7]. As such, persons should address cumulative childhood stress because doing so is paramount to thriving in adulthood.

Participants in The Family: People Helping People Project are traumatized and therefore engage in at-risk behaviors. The authors hypothesized that these at-risk behaviors can be co-morbid with various physical diseases, which could increase the risk of dis-socialization. Traumatization is counteracted when persons participate in The Family Program, consequently increasing resocialization. The authors also hypothesized that there is a direct correlation between traumatization and violent behavior. That is, as exposure to traumatic events increases, so does exposure to violence. The purpose of this study is to investigate these hypotheses.

2. Method

The authors carried out a prospective study in which five (5) psychological tests were given to 209 participants at 16 Family Groups. The tests included the Beck Depression Inventory (BDI) [8], the Adverse Childhood Experience (ACE) questionnaire [9], a Post-Traumatic Stress Disorder screen [10], the Generalized Anxiety Disorder (GAD-7) Scale [11], and the Allen Resocialization Scale [12]. Participants were also given a baseline survey measuring at-risk behavior and physical disease prevalence. A comparison was made between scores from the five tests and responses to the baseline survey. This was done to measure the effects of trauma on physiological and psychological illness. Participants received informed consent forms which they were required to sign. Authors did not attain Institutional Review Board (IRB) approval because the methods of this study involved minimal to no risk to the participants. However, the ethical standards of research in the Bahamas were adhered to.

The researcher, therapist and therapist facilitator all assisted with administering the tests. Participants were offered no incentives for participating in this study. All data were collected and analyzed by the authors during a five (5) month period (November 2019–March 2020).

3. Results and discussion

There were 209 participants in this study. Sixty-three percent (63%) (n = 132) of the participants were female and 37% (n = 77) were male. Due to the adolescent component of the program, the participants less than or equal to 19 years (23%) (n = 48) were almost equally represented with those who were 50–59 years (22%) (n = 46). Seventeen percent (17%) (n = 36) of the participants were 60 years and older. Eleven percent (11%) (n = 22) of the participants was 20–29 years, 13% (n = 28) was 30–39 years and 14% (n = 29) was 40–49 years. A third of the participants graduated from college/university (31%) (n = 65). Twenty-two percent (22%) (n = 47) had some secondary school education, 21% (n = 44) graduated from secondary school and another 21% (n = 43) had attained some college/university education. Three percent (3%) (n = 7) of the participants reported their highest level of education was primary school, and 1% (n = 3) reported having no formal education. More than half (56%) (n = 116) of the participants grew up in a middle-class neighborhood. Thirteen percent (13%) (n = 27) grew up in poverty, 17% (n = 36) lower middle class and 11% (n = 23) upper middle class. Only 3% (n = 7) of the participants grew up in a wealthy neighborhood. Concerning the prevalence of violence in the community, 59% (n = 123) of participants know 1–10 persons who was killed violently. Nineteen percent (19%) (n = 40) of participants know more than 11 persons violently killed. Ten percent (10%) (n = 21) of participants know 31 or more persons violently killed (**Figure 1**), illustrating the severity of the trauma and violence in the country. Regarding the incidence of violent crime (rape, murder, etc.) that occur within the community in an average week, 52% (n = 108) of participants said there were no incidences of violent crime that occur within their community per week. Forty-four percent (44%) (n = 92) of participants indicated there were 1–10 incidences, and 4% (n = 9) indicated there were more than 11 incidences. Regarding the incidences of burglary that occur within the community in an average week, 44% (n = 93) of participants indicated there were no incidences, 49% (n = 102) indicated there were 1–10 incidences and 6% (n = 12) indicated there were more than 11 incidences. One percent (1%) (n = 2) of the participants were unsure how many incidences of burglary occur within their community per week (see **Figure 1**). A third of the participants (32%) (n = 66) have been in The Family Program for 3 months or less. Eleven percent (11%) (n = 22) of the participants have been in the program for 4–6 months, 12% (n = 26) for 7 months to 1 year, and 19% (n = 39) for 1–2 years. Almost a third (27%) (n = 56) of them have been in the program for 3 years or more.

The Beck Depression Inventory (BDI) [8] was given to participants. Results indicate that 45% (n = 94) of participants have normal ups and downs, 18% (n = 38) have a mild mood disturbance, and 9% (n = 18) have borderline clinical depression. Ten percent (10%) (n = 21) of participants were not depressed (they scored zero on

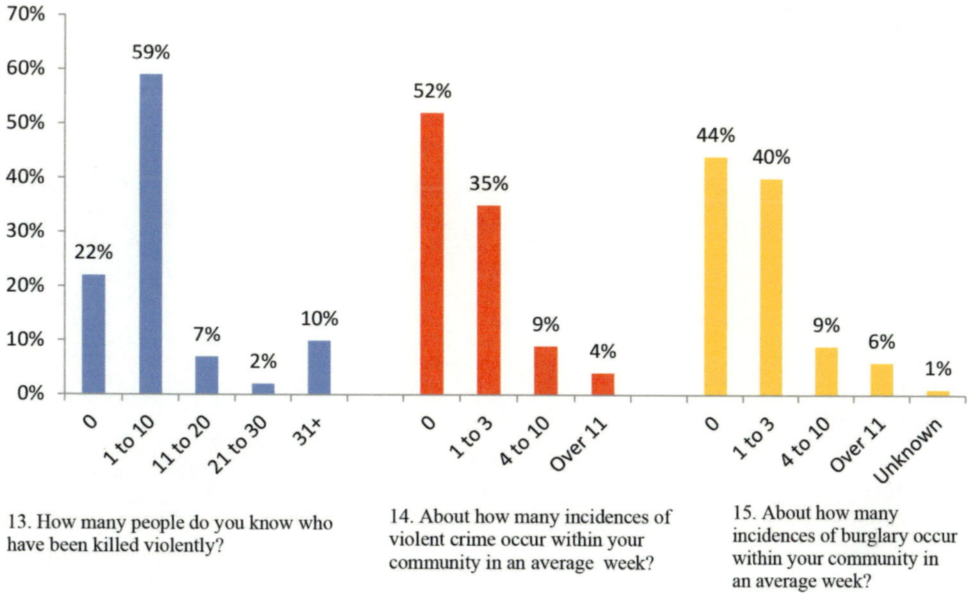

Figure 1.
Prevalence of violence in the community.

the BDI). Eleven percent (11%) (*n* = 22) of the participants have moderate depression and 7% (*n* = 16) have severe/extreme depression.

A 10-item questionnaire measuring adverse childhood experiences (ACE) [9] was given to participants. Any score greater than three (3) is significant. The higher the score, the greater the impact of life experiences [13]. The results indicate that 91 of the participants (44%) scored four (4) or higher on the ACE questionnaire (see **Table 1**).

To further investigate the incidence of physical abuse in childhood, question two of the ACE [9] was analyzed "Did a parent or other adult in the household often push, grab, slap or throw something at you or ever hit you so hard that you had marks or were injured?". Forty-four (44%) (*n* = 93) of participants answered 'yes' to this question. That is, almost half of the participants were physically abused before the age of 18 years. Punishment can easily turn into abuse, especially when anger is involved. Question three of the ACE [9] was analyzed to ascertain the incidence of sexual abuse in childhood. Question three asked "Did an adult or person at least 5 years older than you ever touch or fondle you or have you touch their body in a sexual way or try to or actually have oral, anal or vaginal sex with you?" Twenty-three percent (23%) (*n* = 48) of participants answered 'yes' to this question. That is, almost one-quarter of the participants were sexually abused before the age of 18 years.

Moreover, 23% (*n* = 48) of participants had a history of sexual abuse before the age of 18, and moderate/severe PTSD. If sexual abuse is the only adverse childhood experience a person has, moderate/severe PTSD in adulthood may still occur. Sexual offenses that transpired in the United Kingdom were prosecuted 40 years later, proving the length of time it can take for a victim to come forward. As such, victims can spend years living with the unresolved trauma of sexual abuse [14].

The Post-Traumatic Stress Disorder (PTSD) self-test [10] was given to participants. Authors edited the original questionnaire to make it more understandable to our cohort. The results indicated that 16% (*n* = 33) of the participants did not have PTSD, while 84% (*n* = 176) had moderate or severe PTSD. Participants with moderate or severe PTSD will display symptoms associated with it, which include flashbacks, murderous rage, poor impulse control, and hopelessness [15, 16]. Persons with PTSD can also be destructive. Given the prevalence of violence in the community (see **Figure 1**),

ACE Score	# of Participants
0	30
1	37
2	25
3	26
4	23
5	22
6	20
7	14
8	4
9	5
10	3

Table 1.
Adverse childhood experiences (ACE) scores.

it is not surprising that 84% of participants present with moderate/severe PTSD as PTSD can be triggered by witnessing or experiencing a terrifying event, such as murder [17]. Moreover, with 44% of the participants having a significant amount (four or more) of adverse childhood experiences (see **Table 1**), it is reasonable that 84% of participants would present with moderate/severe PTSD as PTSD may start within 1 month of the event but sometimes may not appear until years after [17]. Forty-one percent (41%) (n = 86) of participants had a significant ACE score and moderate/severe PTSD.

A Generalized Anxiety Disorder Scale (GAD-7) [11] was given to participants. Twenty-three percent (23%) (n = 48) of the participants did not have anxiety, 28% (n = 58) had minimal anxiety, and 23% (n = 48) had mild anxiety. Twenty-six percent (26%) (n = 55) of participants had moderate/severe anxiety. This phenomenon has been common in our work, where people who have murderous rage describe feeling more angry than anxious.

The Allen Resocialization Scale was given to participants. This scale defines resocialization based on many established constructs of personal growth. It is comprised of eight subscales that measure well-being, spirituality, awareness, resilience, stress management, friendliness, self-protection, and family bonds [12]. Six percent (6%) (n = 12) of participants scored 'excellent', 59% (n = 123) scored 'good' and 33% (n = 69) scored 'average'. Only 2% (n = 5) of participants scored 'fair'. No participants scored 'poor' (see **Table 2**). These results indicate that 98% of the participants are resocialized (defined by either an excellent, good, or average score). Since resocialization is the ultimate goal of The Family: People Helping People Program, these results signify a 98% success rate.

Felitti et al. [7] compared ACE scores and patients' reports of at-risk behaviors and disease. There was a graded relationship between the number of adverse experiences in childhood and all 10 risk behaviors (including depression, suicide attempts, substance abuse, etc.) [7, 13]. In this study, the physiological illnesses coded for and used to compare the ACE scores to include: heart disease, cancer, stroke, chronic bronchitis/emphysema, elevated or low cholesterol, elevated blood pressure, diabetes, rheumatism (arthritis), and sexually transmitted disease. At-risk behaviors included alcoholism, regular consumption of alcohol, drug abuse, and regular consumption of drugs. Results indicate that (47%) (n = 98) of the participants had at least one physiological illness. While only 6% (n = 12) responded 'yes' to alcoholism, 32% (n = 67) admitted to regularly consuming alcohol. Nine percent (9%) (n = 19) responded 'yes' to drug abuse, while 23% (n = 48) admitted to regularly using drugs (see **Table 3**). Drugs of choice included marijuana (71%) (n = 34), tobacco (40%) (n = 19), cocaine (10%) (n = 5), ecstasy (4%) (n = 2), and other (often further described as use of

Allen Resocialization Scale Category	# of Participants
Excellent	12
Good	123
Average	69
Fair	5
Poor	0

Table 2.
Allen resocialization scale scores.

Physiological illness/at-risk behavior	# of Participants
Heart disease	23
Cancer	4
Stroke	7
Chronic bronchitis/emphysema	98
Elevated or low cholesterol	44
Elevated blood pressure	62
Diabetes	14
Rheumatism (arthritis)	18
Sexually transmitted disease	10
Alcoholism	12
Regular consumption of alcohol	67
Drug abuse	19
Regular consumption of drugs	48

Table 3.
Physiological illnesses and at-risk behaviors.

medications) (21%) (n = 10). Some participants admitted to the regular consumption of more than one drug. Twenty-three percent (23%) (n = 48) of participants had a significant ACE score and physiological illness. Twenty-one percent (21%) (n = 43) of participants had a significant ACE score and at-risk behavior, defined by alcohol and/or drug abuse.

The self-protection subscale of the Allen Resocialization Scale [12] was used to assess the suicidality of participants. Fifty-eight percent (58%) (n = 121) of participants scored 'excellent', 20% (n = 42) scored 'good', 17% (n = 35) scored 'average' and 5% (n = 11) scored 'poor'.

Suicidal ideations and attempts were measured using question #26 from the baseline questionnaire, which asks,

> Have you ever experienced thoughts of suicide? YES or NO
> Have you ever attempted suicide? YES or NO

Forty percent (40%) (n = 83) of participants had suicidal ideation and 21% (n = 43) had previously attempted suicide. Almost one quarter of participants (24%) (n = 51) had a significant ACE score, moderate/severe PTSD and a history of suicidality (defined as either having a low self-protection score, previous suicidal ideation, or suicide attempt).

Resilience of participants in this study was measured using the Allen Resocialization Scale [12] which includes a resilience subscale. Sixty-three percent (63%) (n = 132) of participants scored either 'excellent' or 'good', 37% (n = 77) scored either 'average' or 'poor'. Eighteen percent (18%) (n = 38) of participants had low resilience (defined as a score of 'average' or 'poor' on the resilience scale), a significant ACE score and moderate/severe PTSD.

In keeping with Dorothy Lewis' hypothesis that the perpetrators (of violence) were once victims themselves [18, 19], we investigated how many of our participants who admitted to being perpetrators of violence were once victims (defined by a significant ACE score or a 'yes' response to questions 27, 28, or 29 of the baseline questionnaire). In our sample, 17% (n = 36) of participants had a significant ACE score and a history of being a perpetrator of violence. Eleven percent (11%) (n = 24) had a history of being a victim and perpetrator of bullying. Thirteen percent (13%) (n = 27) had a history of being a victim and a perpetrator of a violent attack. Five percent (5%) (n = 11) had a history of being a victim and perpetrator of intimate partner violence.

4. Case vignettes

1. A female inmate shared she was incarcerated for fighting the police. When asked if she remembers always being so angry, she became emotional. She explained that her mother was very poor and it was really hard her whole life. She admitted to prostituting herself. Two other inmates said their story was the same. It is important to note that there were only six participants in this session, which means that 50% of them had prostituted themselves because of financial lack. The facilitator noted that the women in this group had many relationships with men where love was not the connection. Instead, anger/violence, a way of expressing emotion, is a powerful form of their communication.

2. A young man presented to one of the groups. He shared that he grew up in a religious home but had issues with his [step] father. His parents were married but divorced before he was born. He had a good stepfather. His mother died when he was 17 years old. He was introduced to sex from the age of four and described being molested by a pastor. He continued the cycle of abuse by sexually abusing his sister from age seven onwards.

3. A female inmate admitted to being imprisoned for murder. She started sessions with The Family Program 2 years ago, at which time she presented as tough, guarded, and seemingly unremorseful. Now, she seems to have grown immensely. She described the sequence of events preceding the incident, her responsibility in it, the warnings of her mother and the impact of leaving her child behind. She admitted that being with her friends was priority. She is now a comforter to new inmates. She believes that being incarcerated may have saved her life. If she had not come to prison, she may have been dead. The facilitator noted that it was riveting to hear the process of murder, which was preceded by a verbal altercation that escalated into a physical confrontation. Despite the incident being an intentional brawl, the perpetrator did not seem to realize murder would be the end result. Before the session ended, the participant shared that when she was 12, she witnessed her brother's murder. It seems that she became detached from that day on. This aloofness eventually led to murder. This is an example of how a hurt child can become a dangerous adult, that is, how the perpetrator was once a victim herself.

5. Conclusion

As the Adverse Childhood Experiences (ACE) studies show [7], early physical and sexual child abuses produces deep shame that is lodged in the unconscious life of the person. This relational trauma and its accompanying dysregulation block the child from flourishing and enjoying life. It impedes their ability to grieve, express deep feelings of commitment, and appreciate simple experiences of joy. In essence, it destroys the child's ability to thrive.

In our sample, 44% (n = 91) of the participants had a significant ACE score, 84% (n = 176) had moderate/severe PTSD and 41% (n = 86) had both a significant ACE score and moderate/severe PTSD. This means that during their time in The Family Program (1–6 or more years), these persons should have had severe violent acting out manifested as domestic violence, murder, suicide or destructive/abusive relationships. Instead, 98% (n = 204) of the participants in this sample who are traumatized and involved in The Family Program scored 'excellent', 'good' or 'average' on the Allen Resocialization Scale [12]. Without The Family Program, these participants may have been 'poorly' resocialized, wreaking havoc in the society. This shows some preliminary evidence that The Family support groups are a protective factor. Despite being traumatized in early childhood, participating in a Family support group can help you change your mind, which will change your life and eventually change your world.

Since this study was completed in March 2020, the COVID-19 pandemic started. Its associated restrictions led to closure of our groups, as we were not allowed to have any gatherings. This has had a detrimental effect on our participants. Many have expressed feeling depressed since not being able to meet. Some have struggled with suicidal ideations and some have attempted suicide. This phenomenon verifies the impact of The Family Group intervention, especially as it relates to providing support for the participants.

6. Limitations

1. On baseline questionnaire 22c, bronchitis is characterized with cough, cold, influenza, pharyngitis, tonsillitis, asthma, etc. As a result, a 'yes' response could have been to any one of these illnesses and not specifically bronchitis, therefore skewing the data. Same is true of question 22p, in terms of coding for diabetes.

2. Baseline questionnaire 20 asks the participant about regular consumption of various substances. However, it was never defined how many times per day/month/week should be considered 'regular consumption'.

7. Software

Data were entered into Microsoft Excel and analyzed in a database created in Microsoft Access.

Acknowledgements

We acknowledge the therapists and the facilitators of the group sessions because without their support and efforts, this work would not have been possible. We also acknowledge all our participants in the program and commend them for taking the courage to embark on their journey to wholeness.

Funding details

This work is supported by the Templeton World Charity Foundation under Grant TWCF 0172.

Disclosure statement

Both authors declare that there were no conflicts of interest regarding this study. Both authors had access to the data at all times, and each had a role in writing the manuscript.

Author details

Keva Bethell* and David Allen
Allen Institute of Research and Training, Nassau, Bahamas

*Address all correspondence to: keva.y.bethell@gmail.com

References

[1] Jekel JF, Allen DF, Podlewski H, Clarke N, Dean-Patterson S, Cartwright P. Epidemic free-base cocaine abuse. Case study from the Bahamas. Lancet. 1986;**1**(8479):459-462

[2] Allen DF, Jekel JF. Crack: The Broken Promise. London: MacMillan Academic and Professional Ltd.; 1991

[3] Bethell K, Allen D, Allen Carroll M. Using a supportive group process to cope with the trauma of social fragmentation and promote re-socialization in the Bahamas. Emergency Medicine: Open Access. 2015;**5**(244). DOI: 10.4172/2165-7548.1000244

[4] Abernethy AD, Allen DF, Allen Carroll M. Adapting group therapy to address real world problems: Insights from groups offered in the Bahamas. International Journal of Group Psychotherapy. 2017;**68**(1):17-34. DOI: 10.1080/00207284.2017.1335582

[5] Allen D, Mayo M, Allen Carroll M, Manganello J, Allen V, Singh J. Cultivating gratitude: Contemplative discovery pathway theory applied to group therapy in the Bahamas. Journal of Trauma & Treatment. 2014;**3**(197). DOI: 10.4172/2167-1222.1000197

[6] Burke-Harris N. The Deepest Well: Healing the Long-Term Effects of Childhood Adversity. New York: Mariner Books; 2018

[7] Felitti V, Anda R, Nordenberg D, Williamson D, Spitz A, Edwards V, et al. Relationship of childhood abuse and household dysfunction to many of the leading causes of death in adults. The adverse childhood experiences (ACE) study. American Journal of Preventive Medicine. 1998;**14**(4):245-258. DOI: 10.1016/s0749-3797(98)00017-8

[8] Beck AT, Ward CH, Mendelson M, Mock J, Erbaugh J. An inventory for measuring depression. Archives of General Psychiatry. 1961;**4**:561-571

[9] Adverse Childhood Experience (ACE) Questionnaire. Available from: https://www.ncjfcj.org/sites/default/files/Finding%20Your%20ACE%20Score.pdf [Retrieved: June 2017]

[10] Post-Traumatic Stress Disorder Self-Test. Available from: https://adaa.org/screening-posttraumatic-stress-disorder-ptsd [Retrieved: June 2017]

[11] Spitzer R, Kroenke K, Williams J, Lowe B. A brief measure for assessing generalized anxiety disorder. Archives of Internal Medicine. 2006;**166**(10):1092-1097. DOI: 10.1001/archinte.166.10.1092

[12] Allen D, Allen-Carroll M, Bethell K, Manganello J. An instrument for assessment of longitudinal community resocialization through a group process intervention. Journal of Trauma & Treatment. 2017;**6**(355). DOI: 10.4172/2167-1222.1000355

[13] Reavis JA, Looman J, Franco KA, Rojas B. Adverse childhood experiences and adult criminality: How long must we live before we possess our own lives? The Permanente Journal. 2013;**17**(2):44-48. DOI: 10.7812/TPP/12-072

[14] BBC News. Savile and Hall: BBC 'Missed Chances to Stop Attacks'. 25 February 2016. Available from: http://www.bbc.com/news/uk-35658398 [Retrieved: 24 April 2020]

[15] George DT, Berger L. Untangling the Mind: Why We Behave the Way We Do. New York: HarperCollins Publishers; 2013

[16] Walkup JT, Rubin DH. Social withdrawal and violence—Newtown, Connecticut. New England Journal of Medicine. 2013;**368**(5):399-401. DOI: 10.1056/NEJMp1215605

[17] Mayo Foundation for Medical Education and Research. Mayo Clinic; 1998. Available from: https://www.mayoclinic.org/diseases-conditions/post-traumatic-stress-disorder/symptoms-causes/syc-20355967 [Retrieved: 27 March 2020]

[18] Lewis DO. From abuse to violence: Psychophysiological consequences of maltreatment. Journal of the American Academy of Child and Adolescent Psychiatry. 1992;**31**(3):383-391. DOI: 10.1097/00004583-199205000-00001

[19] Lewis DO. Guilty by Reason of Insanity: A Psychiatrist Probes the Minds of Killers. New York: Ivy Books; 1998

Chapter 2

Developmental Trauma through a Public Health Lens: The Economic Case for the Developmental Trauma Disorder Diagnosis and a Trauma-informed Vision

Elena Acquarini, Vittoria Ardino and Rosalba Rombaldoni

Abstract

Developmental trauma is a hidden pandemic leading to a multilayered array of negative outcomes across the lifespan, including critical health conditions and increased healthcare utilization. Such a scenario represents a major socio-economic burden with costs for health and social care and for society as a whole. A trauma-informed public health approach puts childhood adversities at the core of treatment and service provision. The chapter firstly outlines how a trauma-informed public health approach embedding the recognition of the Developmental Trauma Disorder diagnosis represents a major shift in conceptualizing health and social care provision and to recognizing the pervasiveness of adverse experiences. Secondly, the chapter elaborates a projective cost analysis to illustrate how the societal, health, and social care costs would be reduced if trauma-related policies were implemented. A multi-disciplinary view—which includes an economic case aspect—could strengthen ACEs prevention efforts and could raise awareness about the problem.

Keywords: child abuse, trauma-informed approach, public health, economic costs, health policy, Developmental Trauma Disorder

1. Introduction

Developmental trauma is a multilayered and cumulative form of trauma, usually of an interpersonal and abusive nature representing serious psychosocial, medical, and policy issues for both the victims and the society. Global community surveys show high prevalence rates of physical (22.9%), emotional (29.1%), and sexual (9.6%) abuse, as well as physical (16.6%) and emotional neglect (18.4). Through a comparison of a series of meta-analyses, Stoltenborgh and colleagues [1] found the overall estimated prevalence rate for CSA to be 12.7–7.6% among boys and 18% among girls globally. For this reason, billions of children are under the attention of the child welfare system for abuse and neglect; daily, services deal with the sequelae of childhood trauma, that often persist for decades [2] and intergenerationally [3] with long-lasting effects on child's neurodevelopment, relationships, learning, and health [4, 5].

Children who have been exposed to interpersonal and chronic stress and trauma develop a broad spectrum of psychopathological outcomes—beyond the most known PTSD clusters that do not fully capture the impact of trauma on children who have been exposed to ongoing danger, disruptive caregiving, and difficult attachment systems. Consequently, most children with trauma-related psychopathology go undetected and do not have access to appropriate treatment.

The chapter addresses the unmet needs of traumatized children within a public health framework. Such a framework elaborates on three interrelated aspects—(1) the importance of the proposed new diagnosis of Developmental Trauma Disorder [6] to identify the complex clinical presentation of long-lasting consequences of child adversities; (2) the need for a universal trauma-informed policy to sustain prevention and treatment of childhood trauma within the systems of care; and (3) cost reductions as a consequence of less misdiagnosis or underdiagnosis leading to ineffective treatment and overload of public services, criminal justice systems, and hospitals [7].

2. The adverse childhood experiences study and the origin of a public health approach to childhood trauma

The so-called "ACEs study" uncovered the public health burden of childhood trauma. The investigation was a major retrospective study involving 17,337 middle-aged, middle-class adults, matching their biomedical and mental health, social function against 10 categories of adverse childhood experiences during infancy, childhood, or adolescence [8]. The authors explained this association as an indirect relationship between stressful conditions and mortality risk factors, including health-related behaviors. The underlying hypothesis was that "stressful or traumatic childhood experiences" have negative neurodevelopmental impacts that persist across development and lifespan and that increase the risk of a variety of health and social problems [8]. The ACEs study reported associations between adversity and lung cancer [9], risk of suicide [10], depressive disorders [11], and ischemic heart disease [12], amongst other effects. Meta-analyses have now been conducted to examine the consistency of findings [13, 14]. Hughes and colleagues [13] conducted a meta-analysis of 37 studies measuring associations between multiple ACEs and health outcomes. Their analysis supported substantially increased health risks to adults who reported multiple exposures to childhood trauma.

The impact on the body's adaptive systems when faced with toxic stress and adverse childhood experiences can lead to allostatic load and extreme behavioral and physiological reactions [15]. In addition, traumatized children develop over time an attentional bias toward the threat, threat sensitization, and heightened stress reactivity, modifying their ability to engage in the cognitive appraisal process, described by Lazarus and Folkman [16] as important to coping. Multiple dangerous events may also appear to be a greater threat unless there is also an appraisal of adequate inner and outer resources to respond to the events. These mind-body processes, taking place across development within person-environment interactions, help to explain some of the correlations between early adversity and later-life health challenges, as well as why the accumulation of risks can increase the likelihood of more risks.

The prevalence of adverse childhood experiences (ACEs) was found to be so common, once they were routinely assessed in clinical practice, and their powerful, dose-related relationship to various damaging outcomes was found to be so strong, that one can only wonder why the relationship of life experiences in the developmental years to adult functionality, disease, and life span was not recognized long ago. Probably, there is a taboo to openly talk about childhood sexual abuse and other forms of maltreatment by parents, thus effectively blocking our ability to detect and fully understand certain difficult and intractable public health problems. Furthermore, there is the potential for a "public health paradox"—many health issues are attempted and unconscious personal coping strategies to handle problems the system cannot comfortably detect leading to increased costs for individuals, healthcare, and the whole society [17–20].

A public health policy approach that is only oriented to treating specific health outcomes, or to changing health risk behaviors—that are also coping mechanisms—cannot sustain effective strategies as it focuses on taking away an attempted solution to deal with problems related to major long-term risks without unacknowledging short-term benefits. For example, people often continue to smoke even when public health policies make it complicated and even after the onset of smoking-related symptoms and illness [21]. A better knowledge of adverse childhood experiences and mind-body coping processes can inform policies to support families and individual development. For example, the American Academy of Pediatrics (AAP) [22] released a Technical Report and Policy Statement on Childhood Toxic Stress [23, 24]. The documents guide ethical action to address and prevent childhood adversities and include language about the importance of screening for ACEs and trauma. Furthermore, the social science literature suggests that preventing and treating child abuse and neglect requires comprehensive research, assessment, and treatment involving professionals across practice fields offering early intervention to at-risk families in school, medical, and other program settings.

In line with this view, a more effective policy framework should include a trauma-informed perspective and the newly proposed diagnosis of Developmental Trauma Disorder to strengthen the strategies to tackle and address the impact of adverse childhood experiences both in clinical and preventive actions.

3. A trauma-informed perspective and the new diagnosis of Developmental Trauma Disorder

Partially informed by ACE science, the underlying principles of the Trauma-Informed-Care paradigm attempt to respond to the aforementioned public health paradox [25]. Such principles include—realizing that trauma is widespread; recognizing symptoms of trauma; responding without further escalation and re-traumatization. The trauma-informed approach recognizes the need for ACEs and trauma screening and then a more focused follow-up assessment without labeling, or judging, but providing a new perspective to understanding the human experience when impacted by trauma.

Public health action often requires a rapid, yet careful response to the available evidence [26]. In the case of ACEs, the real threat is not taking action, given the known short-term and long-term consequences of childhood trauma. While it is true that research is needed to identify evidence-based interventions to address and prevent ACEs, it may take time to realize. It will be imperative that ACEs science be incorporated into medical and allied health training to better prepare future generations of practitioners. Second, we need to conceptualize universal ACEs screening not as a diagnostic tool, but as a powerful surveillance tool that can transform the healthcare culture to be more trauma-informed. Thus, ACEs data can increase recognition that trauma is widespread and associated with numerous health problems across different clinical settings and patient populations.

Many victims of neglect, child abuse, and maltreatment live on the edge of society and depend on social services for most of their lives. Failures at school and in youth welfare institutions are common. Several studies have addressed the enormous healthcare costs arising from traumatization, as described in the following paragraphs, such as medical treatment costs, early retirement, inability to work, need for social benefits, and even imprisonment. If the consequences of childhood traumatization were better detected and represented in the official diagnostic systems, this would assist patients in obtaining compensation and legal support (court, victim aid) and more appropriate treatment.

The conceptualization of Developmental Trauma Disorder attempts to address the point with a specific focus on the mental health consequences and with the goal of providing more possibilities for adequate treatment of childhood trauma. Many abused children do not meet the criteria for a PTSD diagnosis [27]; conversely, DTD captures the complex combination of symptoms and traits of child traumatization by adopting a transdiagnostic model. Van der Kolk and colleagues [28] proposed diagnostic criteria organized into three clusters in addition to the defined symptoms of PTSD—symptoms of emotional and physiological regulation/dissociation; problems with conduct and attention regulation; and difficulties with self-esteem regulation and in managing social connections. Chronic activation of neurobiological systems involved in the regulation of stress and emotion appears to potentiate activation of the relevant neurotransmitters and neuroendocrinological systems. This has also been implicated in severe emotional dysregulation [29, 30]. Several studies reported clear differences in the aptitude of children with and without trauma in regulation and recognition of emotion [31–33]. Individuals with emotion regulation vulnerabilities react faster and more fiercely to emotional stimuli and require more time to calm down after an emotional reaction. This was particularly evident in studies with adult borderline patients [34–36]. Moreover, negative emotional reactions in everyday life seem to be more easily triggered in those patients [37–38]—see **Table 1** below for the DTD diagnostic criteria [39].

Symptoms clusters extend the symptoms of PTSD [40] and follow the structure of CPTSD diagnostic criteria in the 11th revision of the *International Classification of Diseases* [41, 42]. However, DTD–compared to CPTSD diagnosis—embraces the developmental psychology of childhood and adolescence (e.g., assessing self-other boundary confusion and reactive aggression, negative self-appraisals, and relational detachment). Although DTD was proposed as a diagnosis in the fifth edition of the *Diagnostic and Statistical Manual of Mental Disorders DSM-5* [43], it was rejected due to a lack of empirical evidence at that time. However, evidence of the construct validity and its utility for differentiating clinical features from PTSD were supported by emerging studies [44].

First of all, there is substantial evidence indicating that traumatized children are at risk for developing all types of biopsychosocial dysregulations—as outlined in DTD—in addition to, and in the absence of, PTSD [4] and that the polysymptomatic outlook of these children cannot be accounted for fully by PTSD or other psychiatric disorders [45, 46] in addition to the clinical utility of the proposed diagnosis [47]. In a study aiming to test the face validity of DTD by surveying clinicians, Developmental Trauma Disorder symptoms rated as distinguishable from PTSD were—impaired positive and negative affect, affect tolerance and expression, emotion regulation, and

Criteria	Subcriteria
Criterion A: lifetime contemporaneous exposures to both types of developmental trauma	A1: traumatic interpersonal victimization A2: traumatic disruption in attachment bonding with the primary caregiver(s)
Criterion B: current emotion or somatic dysregulation (4 items; 3 required for DTD)	B1: emotion dysregulation B2: somatic dysregulation B3: impaired access to emotion and somatic feelings B4: impaired verbal mediation of emotion or somatic feelings
Criterion C: current attentional or behavioral dysregulation (5 items; 2 required for DTD)	C1: attention bias toward or away from the threat C2: impaired self-protection C3: maladaptive self-soothing C4: non-suicidal self-injury C5: impaired ability to initiate or sustain goal-directed behavior
Criterion D: current relational—or self-dysregulation (6 items; 2 required for DTD)	D1: self-loathing or self-viewed as irreparably damaged and defective D2: attachment insecurity and disorganization D3. betrayal-based relational schemas D4: reactive verbal or physical aggression D5: impaired psychological boundaries D6: impaired interpersonal empathy

Source: Spinazzola et al. [39].

Table 1.
Proposed diagnostic criteria for Developmental Trauma Disorder.

bodily functions and pain. Other Developmental Trauma Disorder symptoms distinguishable from PTSD were—risky behavior, self-harm, self-soothing, impaired physical and emotional boundaries, and expectancy of irresolvable loss. Generally, existing evidence-based treatments were rated as generally effective for only 39% (9 of 23) of the Developmental Trauma Disorder symptoms [48]. Although clinician ratings are not sufficient to validate a diagnosis, they are a guide for indicators mostly used in practice [49]; this study concluded that clinicians considered Developmental Trauma Disorder as distinguishable from PTSD criterion A. In a recent literature review, 21 articles reported the evaluation of DTD symptom criteria using objective, empirical methods (e.g., factor analysis, comorbidity with other diagnostic constructs, associations with trauma exposure type, and clinician ratings of utility). Data supported the DTD construct and its clinical utility with the need for further replication in larger samples [50]. As for the existing investigations, two trials supported the validity of DTD as a unifying diagnosis for traumatized children highlighting the value of putting together a wide spectrum of post-traumatic outcomes and the hope for more effective treatments if this diagnosis was considered [51].

The existence of specific and validated DTD diagnostic criteria may sensitize professionals and the general public to the drastic consequences of child abuse, neglect, and traumatization. Furthermore, children are far more likely to exhibit resilience to childhood trauma when child-serving programs, institutions, and service systems understand the impact of childhood trauma, share common ways to talk and think about trauma, and thoroughly integrate effective practices and policies to address it—an approach often, as explained above, referred to as trauma-informed care (TIC).

4. The economic dimension of adverse childhood experiences

Until recently, little data were available on the economic dimension of ACE-induced costs and the relevant health and social policy issues that are closely related to ACE. The costs to society on this front (specifically trauma follow-up costs) are almost unknown. However, recent studies [52, 53] have estimated the annual economic cost of ACE exposure, relative to 12 between risk factors and causes of ill health,[1] with exorbitant figures for Europe and North America: US$581 billion in the former case (2.7% of GDP) and US$748 billion in the latter case (3.5% of GDP). However, there is a need, despite this large cost dimension, for more detailed data at the national level to implement the development of appropriate policies to prevent the phenomenon.

4.1 The main evidence—Studies from Europe and North America

Although much of the research focuses on the North American area (incidence-based studies) [54, 55], there are studies from an increasing number of countries, including several European countries [56, 57], Australia [58], and Asia [59]. The very recent work by Hughes and colleagues [53] offers an estimate of the annual economic cost attributable to ACE for as many as 28 European countries. It is not the intention of this work to go into the merits of the methodology adopted but to give an assessment of the results obtained. However, some essential methodological features should be recalled—the authors use country-level population attributable fractions (so-called PAFs) for 12 health outcomes attributable to ACEs. They obtain this result from pooled estimates of the possible association between ACEs and health status, and from estimates of the prevalence of ACEs within every single country. Then, for each country, PAFs are applied to the total economic cost for each health outcome, and costs for all outcomes associated with ACEs are summed.

The selection of studies from which the prevalence estimates were extracted was carried out according to specific criteria by the authors [53]. What emerges from the 32 selected studies is an adjusted prevalence value of 37.8%, referring jointly to one and two or more ACEs (**Figure 1**). There are 28 European countries considered. The reported values have an informative function and cannot be assumed to be completely representative of the country. Therefore, a certain amount of care is also required when comparing countries, both because of differences in the methodology used and the characteristics of the sample taken. At the individual country level, the highest value is found in Finland with 69.4%, and the lowest in North Macedonia with 20.4%. When only the adjusted prevalence of two or more ACEs is taken into account, the highest value is again shown by Finland, 38.8%, and the lowest by Greece, 4.2%. Another relevant piece of information from the above-mentioned study concerns the largest shares of PAFs due to ACEs in relation to causes of death—in first place, there is interpersonal violence, followed by harmful use of alcohol, illicit drug use, and anxiety. A low impact is exerted by BMI (body-mass index), for all countries.

[1] The considered risk factors are—harmful alcohol abuse, smoking, illicit drug use, and high BMI (body-mass index); the considered causes of ill health are—depression, anxiety, interpersonal violence, cancer, type 2 diabetes, cardiovascular disease, stroke, and respiratory disease.

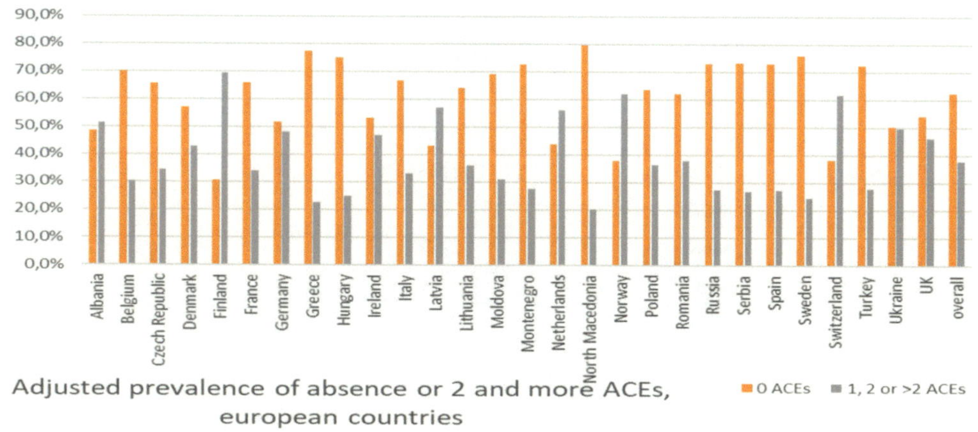

Figure 1.
Adjusted prevalence of adverse childhood experiences. Source: Elaboration of the authors from Hughes et al. [53]. Adjusted ACEs were calculated from available study data.

The following **Table 2** presents ACE-attributable DALYs,[2] the costs associated with all outcomes for each country, together with the level of GDP per capita. The equivalent proportion of GDP is then presented in **Figure 2**.

The range of variation in the number of DALYs attributable to ACEs is quite wide, ranging from low numbers, such as those of Montenegro and North Macedonia (13.0 and 31.6, respectively), to much higher values, such as those of Germany and Russia (2796.6 and 4312.4). The ACE-attributable costs range from 0.2 US$ billion in Montenegro to 129.4 in Germany. Obviously, this evidence cannot be considered directly comparable, as the studies and the samples from which they are derived are quite differentiated in methodologies. However, the analysis of the share absorbed by these costs in terms of GDP is extremely interesting (**Figure 2**): Ukraine, Latvia, and Finland show the highest percentages, with values of 6, 5.5, and 4.1%, Sweden and Turkey with the lowest value, 1.1%. The median proportion among the considered countries is 2.6% and this is also confirmed by other data from another study [60], as shown in **Table 3**, where costs are disaggregated by risk factors and causes of ill health.

The highest rates are for illicit drug use (North America, with 0.80%), smoking and alcohol abuse, in Europe and North America (0.76% in both areas for the former risk factor, 0.65 and 0.34% for the latter). Cardiovascular disease and cancer are the ill health items with the highest costs, again attributable to ACEs, with values around 0.9 and 0.5% for both areas.

The costs outlined appear to be enormous, and underline the importance of investing in a childhood that is safe and has the care and attention it needs. In general, adults exposed to ACEs are more likely to engage in behaviors that are risky to their health and develop physical and mental illnesses that reduce years of healthy working life. The highest proportions in terms of PAFs associated with ACEs are recorded for violence, alcohol abuse, illicit drug use, and mental illness (anxiety and depression). In addition to representing a cost to individuals and society, these outcomes also represent ACEs for the offspring of adults, so one can speak of the intergenerational effects of ACEs [59].

[2] DALYs stands for Disability Adjusted Life Years and expresses the number of years lost due to ill-health, disability or early death.

Country	GDP per capita, US$ 2019	ACE-attributable DALYs (thousands)	ACE-attributable costs (US$ billion)
Albania	5352.9	79.7	0.4
Belgium	46116.7	162.6	7.5
Czech Republic	23101.8	246.5	5.7
Denmark	59822.1	136	8.1
Finland	48685.9	225.2	11
France	40493.9	939.4	38
Germany	46258.9	2796.6	129.4
Greece	19582.5	123.8	2.4
Hungary	16475.7	239.1	3.9
Ireland	78661	97.8	7.7
Italy	33189.6	916.2	30.4
Latvia	17836.4	105	1.9
Lithuania	19455.5	93	1.8
Moldova	4498.5	107.6	0.5
Montenegro	8832	13	0.1
Netherlands	52447.8	536.2	28.1
North Macedonia	6093.1	31.6	0.2
Norway	75419.6	145.7	11
Poland	15595.2	941.5	14.7
Romania	12919.5	660.5	8.5
Russia	11585	4312.4	50
Serbia	7402.4	191.9	1.4
Spain	29613.7	565.9	16.8
Sweden	51610.1	117.9	56.1
Switzerland	81993.7	250.5	20.5
Turkey	9042.5	926.5	8.4
Ukraine	3659	2538.9	9.3
UK	42300.3	1858.7	78.6

Source: Adapted from Hughes et al. [54].

Table 2.
GFP per capita, ACE-attributable DALYs (thousands), and costs (billion) in 28 European countries.

The values reported in terms of cost as a percentage of GDP may plausibly be an underestimate of the true value, because, in addition to the impact on health conditions, there are many other costs at the societal level, such as low educational attainment, unemployment, crime, and other states of social deprivation. The damage is manifested not only in adulthood but also from the earliest stages of life, as children show reduced social and cognitive development, poor school engagement, increased health risks, and juvenile crime. Therefore, the health, as well as social and economic benefits of concrete actions to prevent and contain ACES would materialize much earlier than adult health status (generally considered in studies).

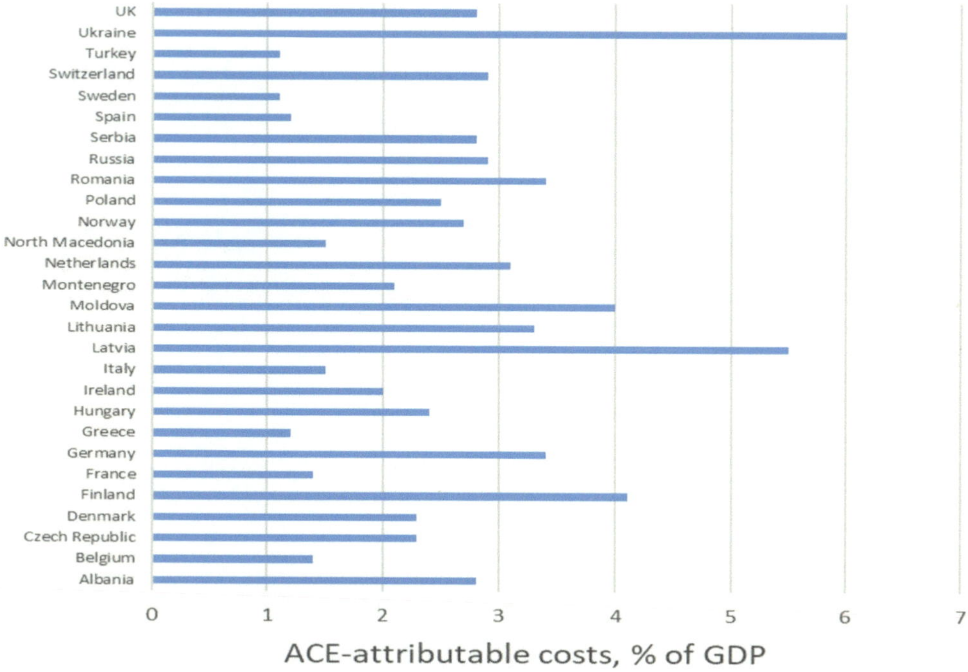

Figure 2.
Adverse childhood experiences attributable costs. Source: Elaboration of the authors from Hughes et al. [53].

With the advent of the pandemic, the conditions predisposing the occurrence of ACEs were exacerbated, and all resilience was lost as children were isolated in traumatic family contexts and all forms of support were cut off. Moreover, the pandemic diverted all resources used in services and activities aimed at preventing ACEs, such as parenting and socio-economic development programs, and youth support services. It is presumable that individuals with ACEs were particularly affected by the pandemic due to their more risky and critical health conditions, which made them vulnerable to severe COVID-19 disease effects, (of a respiratory nature), and other adverse effects associated with the pandemic, such as poor mental health.

Although it is difficult to quantify the differential impact that the pandemic had on people affected and not affected by ACEs, preventive actions in this sense could certainly reduce harmful health behaviors, limit susceptibility to new infections, and thus reduce health risks in the event of future pandemics.

Beyond the limitations that the various studies in terms of the definition of outcome measurements, duration and severity of exposure to ACEs, the possible differences between countries in the association between outcomes and ACEs, the estimates should be interpreted as the best obtainable given the available data. In addition, the considered studies propose a methodology that could be replicated across countries by enhancing the collection of ACE data.

For effective preventive actions, there needs to be uniformity in the approach to both the measurement of ACEs and the methodology. At the European level, ACE studies involving students in 13 countries have been carried out [52], while ACE tools have often been included in routine population health surveys, as in the case of the USA. Critical issues include the use of a narrow range of ACEs events and a simplistic

	Risk factors						Causes of ill health				Total
	Harmful alcohol	**Illicit drug**	**Smoking**	**Obesity**	**Anxiety**	**Depression**	**Cancer**	**Cardiovascular disease**	**Diabetes**	**Respiratory disease**	
Europe	0.65	0.21	0.76	0.18	0.10	0.13	0.54	0.85	0.07	0.21	3.70
North America	0.34	0.80	0.76	0.31	0.17	0.22	0.45	0.92	0.09	0.47	4.53

Source: Adapted from Bellis et al. [58].

Table 3.
Total attributable costs for risk factors/causes of ill health, Europe and North America.

approach to scoring. Certainly, the availability and comparability of evidence and adverse effects related to ACEs could play an important role in gaining political consensus to invest seriously in prevention. Population studies should cover ACEs events and therefore converge on how to measure them and in which population groups.

5. Toward trauma-informed policies

The long-lasting consequences of childhood trauma for individuals and society demonstrate an impact on health and economics. The policy context of ACEs recommends a collection and use of data in a non-diagnostic, multi-generational, trauma-informed, and including assessment of patient resiliency. Ethically speaking, we really cannot afford to wait another 20 years to take the needed action for addressing and preventing ACEs.

The ACE phenomenon is associated with very high health and economic costs, both nationally and internationally. Estimates from various studies indicate a percentage, in terms of GDP, of about 2.6% at the European level and 4.5% for North America. This is, of course, an underestimate, and the more data are available and comparable, the more accurate the value may be. In fact, the costs of ACEs go well beyond ill health, having a strong social and educational impact. The pandemic has further exacerbated inequalities, increased risk factors, and diverted important resources away from prevention and containment.

The other important aspect is the influence that these studies may have on decision-making processes. Even if the estimates presented reflect the health costs associated with ACEs (and presumably health costs are only a part), there would still be an enormous economic burden (even half of the costs associated with ACEs would amount to 0.6% of the GDP of the 28 European countries). Moreover, the total cost of ACEs includes other costs, such as unemployment, youth delinquency, and social deprivation. As stated in other studies [60, 61], early identification of the problem can bring huge savings for the health system, and only a precocious intervention can stop the escalation of all the direct and indirect costs correlated to ACEs.

The COVID-19 pandemic has absorbed excessive resources, yet policymakers cannot reduce spending on ACEs prevention programs. Governments should strive for greater equity in health, and create a resilient population for future pandemics. Many studies show that when society does not care about safe child development, it then incurs very high costs, both individually and in the community. To support this endeavor, a service system transformation, community partnerships are warranted.

The service system can be transformed to support appropriate ACE responses with the recognition of the existence of a Developmental Trauma Disorder for a better pathway to interrupt intergenerational patterns and promote effective interventions and treatments. This is in line with the increased recognition of the need for trauma-informed service [62, 63] with prevention-based programming offered through a variety of means—these are approaches in support of national health policy. For example, bonding to a healthy school environment is connected to reduced health risk behaviors as well as stronger social and academic skills [64]. In these ways, service systems could ideally facilitate community development and offer complementary prevention and intervention services within the local context. Raising awareness and increasing societal support are complementary to clinical interventions designed to support traumatized children.

If effective trauma-informed policies and DTD-based diagnoses are associated with trauma prevention and overall health, this suggests that services may lead to societal cost savings [65, 66]. However, just as there is a need for explicitly trauma-informed prevention and intervention research, there is also a need for empirical cost-effectiveness research on these activities. The cost savings associated with human capital development [67] highlight that effective health and social care practices are a worthwhile investment. The concept of human capital helps to explain the profitability of protecting children from adverse experiences and fostering development within the context of healthy environments and supportive relationships. A number of studies have already identified noteworthy returns from early intervention programs for disadvantaged children [67, 68]. For example, one study by the 2000 Nobelist in Economics, James Heckman, found that by the time a child was 27 years old, there was a return of $5.70 on each dollar spent in childhood, with further returns over time. In addition to these individual returns, society is saved from the expense of programs created to intervene with costly effects of adverse childhood experiences, and other members of society gain from more constructive social relations.

Families, schools, and other systems all contribute to human capital development [69, 70]. Developmental Trauma Disorder within a trauma-informed approach connects activities to National Health Policy through the evident role of a public health vision of trauma in health promotion and disease prevention. Integrating services and developing multidisciplinary DTD teams to streamline and increase service access (especially among disadvantaged communities) and evaluating the policies and programs coordinating these activities should enable clinical intervention, community development, prevention, and services research to protect children from trauma and heal their wounds [71]. Partnering with economists to analyze cost-savings associated with trauma-informed prevention and intervention could also increase the possibilities of raising awareness of the generally hidden problem of adverse childhood experiences and their costs.

There is a need for implementing trauma-informed-care intervention and prevention research that attends to mind-body processes contributing to health, to developmental trauma consequences. Investments in effective child trauma prevention and intervention are likely to save notable human and economic costs.

Author details

Elena Acquarini[1], Vittoria Ardino[2] and Rosalba Rombaldoni[3]*

1 Urbino University, Italian Society for Traumatic Stress Study (SISST), Urbino, Italy

2 Urbino University, Italian Society for Traumatic Stress Study (SISST), European Society for Traumatic Stress Studies (ESTSS), Urbino, Italy

3 Urbino University, Urbino, Italy

*Address all correspondence to: rosalba.rombaldoni@uniurb.it

References

[1] Stoltenborgh M, Bakermans-Kranenburg MJ, Alink LRA, van Ijzendoorn MH. The prevalence of child maltreatment across the globe: Review of a series of meta-analyses. Child Abuse Review. 2015;**24**(1):37-50. DOI: 10.1022/car.2353

[2] Thoma V, Weiss-Cohen L, Filkukova P, Ayton P. Cognitive predictors of precautionary behavior during the COVID-19 pandemic. Frontiers in Psychology. 2021;**12**:589800. DOI: 10.3389/fpsyg.2021.6589800

[3] Greene CA, Haisley L, Wallace C, Ford JD. Intergenerational effects of childhood maltreatment: A systematic review of the parenting practices of adult survivors of childhood abuse, neglect and violence. Clinical Psychology Review. 2020;**80**:101891. DOI: 10-1016/j.cpr.2020.101891

[4] D'Andrea W, Ford JD, Stolbach B, Spinazzola J, van der Kolk BA. Understanding interpersonal trauma in children: Why we need a developmentally appropriate trauma diagnosis. The American Journal of Orthopsychiatry. 2012;**82**(2):187-200. DOI: 10.1111/j.1939-0025.2012.01154.x

[5] Teicher MH, Samson JA. Annual research review: Enduring neurobiological effects of childhood abuse and neglect. Journal of Child Psychology and Psychiatry. 2016;**57**(3):241-266. DOI: 10.1111/jcpp.12507

[6] Spinazzola J, van der Kolk BA, Ford JD. Developmental trauma disorder: A legacy of attachment trauma in victimized children. Journal of Traumatic Stress. 2021;**34**(4):711-720. DOI: 10.1002/jts.22697

[7] Danese A, McLaughlin KA, Samara M, Stover CS. Psychopathology in children exposed to trauma: Detection and intervention needed to reduce downstream burden. BMJ. 2020;**371**:m3073. DOI: 10.1136/bmj.m3073

[8] Felitti VJ, Anda RF, Nordenberg D, Willamson DF, Spitz AM, Edwards V, et al. Relationship of childhood abuse and household dysfunction to many of the leading causes of death in adults: The Adverse Childhood Experiences (ACE) study. American Journal of Preventive Medicine. 1998;**14**(4):245-258. DOI: 10.1016/S0749-3797(98)00017-8

[9] Brown DW, Anda RF, Felitti VJ, Edwards VJ, Malarcher AM, Croft JB, et al. Adverse childhood experiences are associated with the risk of lung cancer. A prospective cohort study. BMC Public Health. 2010;**10**:20. DOI: 10.1186/1471-2458-10-20

[10] Dube SR, Anda RF, Felitti VJ, Chapman DP, Williamson DF, Giles WH. Childhood abuse, household dysfunction and the risk of attempted suicide throughout the life span. Findings from the Adverse Childhood Experiences Study. Journal of the American Medical Association. 2001;**286**(24):3089-3096. DOI: 10.1001/jama.286.24.3089

[11] Chapman DP, Whitfield CL, Felitti VJ, Dube SR, Edwards VJ, Anda RF. Adverse childhood experiences and the risk of depressive disorders in adulthood. Journal of Affective Disorders. 2004;**82**(2):217-225

[12] Dong M, Giles WH, Felitti VJ, Dube SR, Williams JE, Chapman DP, et al. Insights into causal pathways for ischemic heart disease. Circulation. 2004;**110**(3):1761-1766. DOI: 10.1181/01.CIR.0000143074.54995.7F

[13] Hughes K, Bellis MA, Hardcastle KA, Sethi D, Butchart A, Mikton C, et al. The effect of multiple adverse childhood experiences on health: A systematic review and meta-analysis. The Lancet Public Health. 2017;**2**(8):e356-e366. DOI: 10.1016/S2468-2667(17)30118-4

[14] Holman DM, Ports KA, Buchanan ND, Hawkins NA, Merrick MT, Metzier M, et al. The association between Adverse Childhood Experiences and risk of cancer in adulthood: A systematic review of the literature. Pediatrics. 2016;**138**(Suppl. 1):581-591. DOI: 10.1542/peds.2015-4268L

[15] McEwen BS. Redefining neuroendocrinology. Epigenetics of brain-body communication over the life course. Frontiers in Neuroendocrinology. 2018;**49**:8-30. DOI: 10.1016/j.yfrne.2017.11.001

[16] Lazarus RS, Folkman S. Stress, Appraisal and Coping. New York, US: Springer Publishing Company; 1984. p. 445

[17] Fletcher J, Wolfe B. Long-term consequences of childhood ADHD on criminal activities. The Journal of Mental Health Policy and Economics. 2009;**12**(3):119-138

[18] Kendall-Tackett K. The health effects of childhood abuse: Four pathways by which abuse can influence health. Child Abuse & Neglect. 2002;**26**(6-7):715-729. DOI: 10.1016/S0145-2134(02)00343-5

[19] Springer KW, Sheridan J, Kuo D, Carnes M. The long-term health outcomes of childhood abuse. Journal of General Internal Medicine. 2003;**18**: 864-870. DOI: 10.1046/j.1525-1497.2003.20918.x

[20] Norman RE, Byambaa M, De R, Butchart A, Scott J, Vos T. The long-term health consequences of child physical abuse, emotional abuse and neglect: A systematic review and meta-analysis. PLoS Medicine. 2012;**9**(11):e1001349. DOI: 10.1371/journal.pmed.1001349

[21] Edwards VJ, Anda RF, Gu D, Dube SR, Felitti VJ. Adverse childhood experiences and smocking persistence in adults with smoking-related symptoms and illness. The Permanente Journal. 2007;**11**(2):5-13. DOI: 10.7812/tpp/06-110

[22] American Academy of Pediatrics (AAP). 2018. Available from: https://www.aap.org/en-us/advocacy-and-policy/aap-health-initiatives/Screening/Pages/Screening-Tools.aspx

[23] American Academy of Pediatrics (AAP). Policy statement: Early childhood, toxic stress and the role of the pediatrician: Translating developmental science into lifelong health. Pediatrics. 2012a;**129**(1):e232-e246. DOI: 10.1542/peds.2011-2662

[24] American Academy of Pediatrics (AAP). Tecnical report: The lifelong effects of early childhood adversity and toxic stress. Pediatrics. 2012b;**129**(1):e232-e246. DOI: 10.1542/peds.2011-2663

[25] Substance Abuse and Mental Health Services Administration (SAMHSA). 2014. Available from: http://www.samhsa.gov/nctic/trauma-interventions

[26] Public Health Leadership Society. Principles of the ethical practice of public health. 2002. Available from: https://www.alpha.org/media/files/pdf/membergroups/ethic_rochure.ashx

[27] van der Kolk BA. The Body Keeps the Score: Mind, Brain and Body in the

Transformation of Trauma. New York, US: Viking Penguin; 2014. p. 441

[28] van der Kolk BA, Pynoos RS, Cicchetti D, Cloitre M, D'Andrea W, Ford JD, Leberman AF, Putnam FW, Saxe G, Spinazzola J, Stolbach BC, Teicher M. Proposal to include a developmental trauma disorder diagnosis for children and adolescents in DSM-V. Available from: http://www.traumacenter.org/announcements/DTD_papers_Oct_09.pdf

[29] Finkelor D, Vanderminden J, Turner H, Hamby S, Shattuck A. Upset among youth in response to questions about exposure to violence, sexual assault and family maltreatment. Child Abuse & Neglect. 2014;**38**:217-223. DOI: 10.1016/j.chiabu.2013.07.021

[30] Dubowitz H, Feigelman S, Lane W, Kim J. Pediatric primary care to help prevent child maltreatment: The Safe Environment for Every Kid (SEEK) Model. Pediatrics. 2009;**123**:858-864. DOI: 10.1542/peds.2008-1376

[31] Meehan AJ, Latham RM, Arseneault L, Stahl D, Fisher HL, Danese A. Developing an individualized risk calculator for psychopathology among young people victimized during childhood: A population-representative cohort study. Journal of Affective Disorders. 2020;**262**:90-98. DOI: 10.1016/j.ad.2019.10.034

[32] Walden TA, Smith MC. Emotion regulation. Motivation and Emotion. 1997;**21**(1):7-25

[33] Mavranezouli I, Megnin-Viggars O, Trickey D, Meiser-Stedman R, Daly C, Dias S, et al. Cost-effectiveness of psychological interventions for children and young people with post-traumatic stress disorder. Journal of Child Psychology and Psychiatry. 2020;**61**:699-710. DOI: 10.1111/jcpp.13142

[34] McLaughlin KA, Colich NL, Rodman AM, Wiessman DG. Mechanisms linking childhood trauma exposure and psychopathology: A transdiagnostic model of risk and resilience. BMC Medicine. 2020;**18**:96. DOI: 10.1186/s12916.020.01561.6

[35] Schore AN. Effect of early relational trauma on affect regulation: The development of borderline personality disorders and a predisposition to violence. In: Schore AN, editor. Affect Dysregulation and Disorders of the Self. New York: W.W. Norton; 2003. pp. 266-306

[36] Purgato M, Gross AL, Betancourt T, Bolton P, Bonetto C, Gastaldon C, et al. Focused psychosocial interventions for children in low-resource humanitarian settings: A systematic review and individual participant data meta-analysis. The Lancet Global Health. 2018;**6**:e390-e400. DOI: 10.1016/S2214.109X(18)30046-9

[37] El-Khodary B, Samara M. Effectiveness of a school-based intervention on the student's mental health after exposure to war-related trauma. Frontiers in Psychiatry. 2020;**10**:1031. DOI: 10.3389/fpsyt.2019.01031

[38] Ebner-Priemer UW, Kuo J, Schlotz W, Kleindienst N, Rosenthal MZ, Linean MM, et al. Distress and affective dysregulation in patients with borderline personality disorder: A psychophysiological ambulatory monitoring study. Journal of Nervous and Mental Disorders. 2008;**196**(4):314-320. DOI: 10.1097/NMD.ob013e31816a493f

[39] Spinazzola J, van der Kolk BA, Ford JD. Psychiatric comorbidity of developmental trauma disorder and posttraumatic stress disorder: Findings from the DTD field trial replication (DTDFT-R). European Journal of

Psychotraumatology. 2021;**12**(1):1929028. DOI: 10.1080/20008198.2021.1929028

[40] Ford JD, Spinazzola J, van der Kolk BA, Grasso D. Toward an empirically-based Developmental Trauma Disorder diagnosis for children: Factor structure, item characteristics, reliability and validity of the Developmental Trauma Disorder Semi-Structured interview (DTD-SI). The Journal of Clinical Psychiatry. 2018;**79**(5):e1-e9. DOI: 10.4088/JCP.17m11675

[41] World Health Organization (WHO). International Statistical Classification of Diseases and Related Health Problems. 11th ed. (ICD-11). 2019. Available from: https://icd.who.int/

[42] Haselgruber S, Solva K, Lueger-Schuster B. Symptom structure of ICD-11 Complex Posttraumatic Stress Disorder (CPTSD) in trauma-exposed foster children: Examining the International Trauma Questionnaire-Child and Adolescent Version (ITQ-CA). European Journal of Psychotraumatology. 2020;**11**(1):1818974. DOI: 10.1080/20008198.2020.1818974

[43] American Psychiatric Association APA. Diagnostic and statistical manual of mental disorders, 5th ed. DSM-5. 2013. DOI: 10.1176/appi.books.9780890425596

[44] Spinazzola J, van der Kolk BA, Ford JD. When nowhere is safe: Trauma history antecedents of posttraumatic stress disorder and Developmental Trauma Disorder in childhood. Journal of Traumatic Stress. 2018;**31**(5):631-642. DOI: 10.1002/jts.22320

[45] Ford JD, Fraleigh LA, Albert DB, Connor DF. Child abuse and autonomic nervous system hyporesponsivity among psychiatrically impaired children. Child Abuse & Neglect. 2010;**34**(7):507-515. DOI: 10.1016/j.chiabu.2009.11.005.10

[46] Ford JD, Fraleigh LA, Connor DF. Child abuse and aggression among seriously emotionally disturbed children. Journal of Clinical Child and Adolescent Psychology. 2010;**39**(1):25-34. DOI: 10.1080/15374410903401104

[47] First MB. Clinical utility: A prerequisite for the adoption of a dimensional approach in DSM. Journal of Abnormal Psychology. 2005;**114**(4):560-564. DOI: 10.1037/0021-843X.114.4.560

[48] Ford JD, Grasso D, Greene C, Levine J, Spinazzola J, van der Kolk BA. Clinical significance of a proposed developmental trauma disorder diagnosis: Results of an international survey of clinicians. The Journal of Clinical Psychiatry. 2013;*74*(8):841-849. DOI: 10.4088/JCP.12m08030

[49] Cloitre M, Courtois CA, Charuvastra A, Carapezza R, Stolbach BD, Green BL. Treatment of complex PTSD: Results of the ISTSS expert clinician survey on best practices. Journal of Traumatic Stress. 2011;**24**(6):615-627. DOI: 10.1002/jts.20697

[50] Morelli NM, Villodas MT. A systematic review of the validity, reliability and clinical utility of developmental trauma disorder (DTD) symptom criteria. Clinical Child and Family Psychology Review. 2021

[51] van der Kolk BA, Ford JD, Spinazzola J. Comorbidity of developmental trauma disorder (DTD) and post-traumatic stress disorder: Findings from DTD field trial. EJPT. 2019;**10**(1):1562841. DOI: 10.1080/200008198.2018.1562841

[52] Hughes KE, Bellis M, Sethi D, Andrew R, Yon Y, Wood S, et al. Adverse childhood experiences, childhood relationships and associated substance use and mental health in young Europeans. European Journal of

Public Health. 2019;**29**:741-747. DOI: 10.1093eurpub/ckz037

[53] Hughes K, Ford K, Bellis MA, Glendinning F, Harrison E, Passmore J. Health and financial costs of adverse childhood experiences in 28 European countries. A systematic review and meta-analysis. The Lancet Public Health. 2021;**6**(11):e848-e857. DOI: 10.1016/S2468-2667(21)00232-2

[54] Fang X, Brown DS, Florence CS, Mercy JA. The economic burden of child maltreatment in the United States and implications for prevention. Child Abuse & Neglect. 2012;**36**(2):156-165. DOI: 10.1016/j.chiabu.2011.10.006

[55] Peterson C, Kearns MC, McIntosh WL, Estefan LF, Nicolaidis C, McCollister KE, et al. Lifetime economic burden of intimate partner violence among US adults. American Journal of Preventive Medicine. 2018;**55**(4):433-444. DOI: 10.1016/j.amepre.2018.04.049

[56] Sethi D, Bellis M, Hughes K, Gilbert R, Mitis F, Galea G. European report on preventing child maltreatment. WHO Regional Office for Europe; 2013. Available from: https://apps.who.int/iris/handle/10665/326375

[57] Habetha S, Bleich S, Weidenhammer J, Fegert JM. A prevalence-based approach to societal costs occurring in consequence of child abuse and neglect. Child and Adolescent Psychiatry and Mental Health. 2012;**6**:35. DOI: 10.1186/1753-2000-6-35

[58] McCarthy MM, Taylor P, Norman RE, Pezzullo L, Tucci J, Goddard C. The lifetime economic and social costs of child maltreatment in Australia. Children and Youth Services Review. 2016;**71**:217-226. DOI: 10.1016/j.childyouth.2016.11.014

[59] Fang X, Fry DA, Brown DS, Mercy JA, Dunne MP, Butchart AR, et al. The burden of child maltreatment in the East Asia and Pacific Region. Child Abuse & Neglect. 2015;**42**:146-162. DOI: 10.1016/j.chiabu.2015.02.012

[60] Bellis MA, Hughes K, Ford K, Rodriguez GR, Sethi D, Passmore J. Life course health consequences and associated annual costs of adverse childhood experiences across Europe and North America: A systematic review and meta-analysis. The Lancet Public Health. 2019;**10**:e517-e528. DOI: 10.1016/S2468-2667(19)30145-8

[61] Narayan AJ, Lieberman AF, Masten AS. Intergenerational transmission and prevention of adverse childhood experiences (ACEs). Clinical Psychology Review. 2021;**85**:e101997. DOI: 10.1016/j.cpr.2021.101997

[62] Rombaldoni R. Economic evaluation of child maltreatment: Is there any place for prevention? Maltrattamento e abuso all'infanzia. 2017;**19**:11-29. DOI: 10.3280/MAL2017-002002

[63] Ardino V, Rombaldoni R. Adverse childhood experiences: Healthcare policy and economics implications. Maltrattamento e abuso all'infanzia. 2017;**19**:7-10. DOI: 10.3280/MAL2017-002001

[64] Harris M, Fallot RD. Using Trauma Theory to Design Service Systems. London, UK: Jossey-Bass/Wiley; 2001. p. 120

[65] Finkelstein N, Markoff LS. The Women Embracing Life and Living (WELL) Project: Using the relational model to develop integrated system of care for women with alcohol/drug use and mental health disorders with histories of violence. Alcoholism

Treatment Quarterly. 2005;**22**(3-4): 63-80. DOI: 10.1300/J020v22n03_04

[66] Catalano RF, Haggerty KP, Oesterle S, Fleming CB, Hawkins JD. The importance of bonding to school for healthy development: Findings from the Social Development Research Group. The Journal of School Health. 2004;**74**(7):252-261. DOI: 10.1111/j.1746-1561.2004.tb08281.x

[67] Larkin H, Records J. Adverse childhood experiences: Overview, response strategy and integral theory. Journal of Integral Theory and Practice. 2007;**2**(3):1-25

[68] Larkin H, Felitti VJ, Anda RF. Social work and adverse childhood experiences research: Implications for practice and health policy. Social Work in Public Health. 2014;**29**(1):1-16. DOI: 10.1080/19371918.2011.619433

[69] Heckman JJ, Krueger AB. Inequality in America: What Role for Human Capital Policy? Cambridge - Massachusetts, US: MIT Press; 2003. p. 370

[70] Karoly LA, Kilburb MR, Cannon JS. Early Childhood Interventions: Proven Results, Future Promise. Santa Monica, CA: RAND Corporation; 2005. p. 200. DOI: 10.7249/MG341

[71] Ford JD, Spinazzola J, van der Kolk BA, Chan G. Toward an empirically based Developmental Trauma Disorder diagnosis and semi-structured interview for children: The DTD field trial replication. Acta Psychiatrica Scandinavica. 2022. DOI: 10.1111/acps.13424. Advance online publication. https://doi.org/10.1111/acps.13424

Chapter 3

Childhood Exposure to Violence: Looking through a Life-Course Perspective

Sílvia Fraga, Mariana Amorim and Sara Soares

Abstract

Childhood is the most important period of development during life course, highly sensitive to external influences and with a profound impact on children's well-being. During this period, the foundations for every individual's physical and mental health capacities and attainment are laid, influencing children's lives throughout adolescence, adulthood and aging. Violence is one of the most traumatic experiences that can impact the healthy development of the child, compromising its growth and future health. Although violence assessment in the scope of a cohort study comprises methodological and ethical challenges, a life-course perspective allows researchers to understand the effects of multiple forms of violence by distinguishing between repetitive violence over time and isolated incidents, the occurrence of violent experiences in different contexts and settings, as well as the interconnection between different experiences of trauma. This chapter aims to demonstrate the importance of a life-course perspective to understand the detrimental relationship between early exposure to violence and worse health in the first years of life.

Keywords: violence at home, peer violence, child's violence

1. Introduction

Exposure to violence can have different manifestations throughout the life course, but all forms of violent behaviors share common characteristics: (1) the use of control strategies depriving others of safety, freedom, health and, in extreme cases, life; (2) the magnitude of the problem affecting particularly the most vulnerable groups; (3) the potential for intergenerational transmission; and (4) a smashing impact at different levels of influence, namely individuals, families, neighborhoods, communities, and society [1–4].

Violence can take several forms throughout the life cycle, being an individual's age is an important determinant of the type of violence that people may experience [5]. Therefore, violence has causes, intents, circumstances, and contributing factors that vary according to each individual life cycle stage. Linking together all these events, experiences and behaviors makes it possible to map out developmental pathways from childhood to later ages [5, 6]. With longitudinal studies, it is possible to study continuity and changes occurring in life as they are central to identifying links between distinct phenomena over the life course and thus to describe social processes that both produce and alter developmental trajectories. Such links are essential to understanding the continuity of the experience and behavior, as well as life-course changes that create new states and circumstances that might be unexpected.

Importantly, this concern with the development process includes a wide range of life outcomes [7]. One of the more prominent themes in life-course research is the identification of factors that put one at risk for adversity in later life.

Additionally, violence is a sensitive topic to research, with specific challenges that are different from those that arise when studying other social or health problems. Usually, monitoring systems restrict the occurrence of interpersonal violence to those who seek hospital care or report their experiences to authorities or social support systems [8]. Therefore, researchers who aim to identify and measure violence besides the tip of the iceberg will need to ask people about violent experiences that occur behind closed doors. Even more challenging is when the goal is to study violence in children, where more delicate ethical issues arise, such as obtaining consent for participation in the research that needed to be provided by their own parents; conducting interviews with or administering tests to the children; and providing information about test results to parents or others outside the research team. The research team faces questions as who is responsible for giving consent for children to participate in research, which is further complicated by the potential adversarial relationship between abusing parent and abused child [9].

Among the methodological challenges that should be addressed are the need to explore the effects of multiple forms of maltreatment and the timing, chronicity, and discontinuity of violence episodes. Some children may live in a continually abusive environment, while others may experience only one incident of brief duration [10]. Thus, longitudinal research allows distinguishing between repetitive violence episodes over time and isolated incidents of violence. Moreover, false reporting may not be discarded when we are assessing violence or abuse experiences. However, evidence shows that false allegations of abuse are much less common than the problem of victims who fail to report abuse, and the widespread false denials and minimization of violence by perpetrators, and in general, abuse is vastly under-reported [11]. Also, many of these experiences, especially those suffered by children and women, may remain hidden since perpetrators have an interest in hampering reports and detection.

This chapter aims to demonstrate the importance of a life-course perspective to understand the detrimental relationship between early exposure to violence and worse health in the first years of life.

2. The early exposure to violence

Violence against children includes all forms of violence whether perpetrated by parents or other caregivers, peers, partners, or strangers. This problem is identified as a public health issue and a human rights concern with high social impact, and potentially devastating and costly consequences [12]. Levels of violence against children are extremely high, and it is estimated that, worldwide, up to 1 billion children aged 2–17 years experienced neglect or were victims of physical, sexual, or emotional violence in their lifetime [13].

Childhood is the most important period of development during life course, highly sensitive to external influences and with a profound impact on children's lives [14, 15]. During this period, the foundations for every individual's physical and mental health capacities and attainment are laid, influencing growth, development, and well-being in adolescence and adulthood.

Early life experiences and environments may negatively influence later experiences, opportunities, and health risk factors [16]. Thus, being exposed to violence during childhood and adolescence could be particularly disruptive to normal psychological development when it occurs during these periods [17] and may damage health over time.

The exposure to violent experiences should be approached since the perinatal period.

2.1 Intergenerational effects of maternal exposure to violence

Violence against women may have direct and indirect effects on the children. Intimate partner violence can have significant adverse effects on victims at any time in their life but has special significance during pregnancy because of the added potential harms to the unborn child. The detrimental effects of adverse and negative gestational experiences, including exposure to violence during pregnancy, on many aspects of a child's development, are well described in the literature [18]. Intimate partner violence during pregnancy is associated with poor health outcomes for the fetus, newborn, and infant up to 1 year postpartum [19, 20]. A study conducted in a public maternity of a general Portuguese university hospital showed that one in 10 women reported physical abuse during pregnancy, and almost half of them reported they had suffered severe acts, such as punching, kicking, bruises, cuts, and/or continuing pain, beaten up, severe contusions, broken bones, head, internal, and/or permanent injury [21]. Also, this study showed that reports of physical abuse during pregnancy were significantly associated with preterm delivery (odds ratio (OR) =3.72; 95% confidence interval (95%CI) between 2.59 and 5.33) [21]. Exposure to violence during pregnancy also increases the risk for antepartum hemorrhage, a condition that can be fatal for the unborn [22, 23], increased fetal morbidity [24], intrauterine growth restriction [23], and low birth weight [19].

Being that the womb is a shared environment between mother and infant, maternal experiences can also affect the developing fetus. On one hand, experiences of abuse, occurring either before and during pregnancy, increase the likelihood of abused women being involved in behaviors that may be detrimental to the fetus, including smoking [25], drug use [26, 27], being overweight [28], stress [29], when compared to unexposed women. On the other hand, increased risk of the health outcomes on the child may occur through different pathways: (1) dysregulation of the locus coeruleus-noradrenergic system through the effects of maternal cortisol on epigenetic modification of genes controlling the development of this system [30, 31]); (2) disruption of brain development by impairing placental circulation [32]); (3) dysregulation of the hypothalamic-pituitary-adrenal axis in the fetus [18, 33]; and (4) triggering of developmental immunotoxicity, through autoimmunity or inflammation of myelomonocytic cells in the brain [34]. Depending on the system affected, several outcomes may emerge on the child's health. Prenatal stress may have a lasting impact on the child's behavior, increasing the risk of autism spectrum disorder [35], Attention Deficit Hyperactivity Disorder (ADHD) [36], and worse general intellectual and language functioning [37]. For instance, increased maternal cortisol along with a downregulation of the enzyme 11β-HSD2, which converts cortisol into its inactive form, can lead to changes in behavioral development and make the infant more susceptible to stress later in life [38].

On the other hand, children living in a family where the mother is exposed to violence are frequently abused themselves, and mothers exposed to violence or threats are often insufficient caregivers which could affect the children regardless of whether they have seen the violent act or not [39].

2.2 Violence experiences at home

In 1962, child maltreatment received widespread attention by the medical profession and the general public after Kempe's publication [40]. Kempe described the battered child syndrome, characterized by the clinical manifestations of serious physical abuse in young children, generally inflicted by a parent or a foster parent. In this chapter, Kempe stated that "physicians, because of their feelings and their difficulty in playing a role that they find hard to assume, may have great reluctance in believing that parents were guilty of abuse" [40].

Violence against children perpetrated by adults within the family is one of the least visible forms of child maltreatment, as much of it takes place in the privacy of domestic life. However, this problem is widely prevalent in all societies [41]. Much physical violence against children is inflicted as a punishment, and it is accepted by parents once it is considered by the prevailing social norms as the correct means of discipline. Corporal punishment of children in the form of hitting, punching, kicking, or beating, is socially and legally accepted in some countries [12], being, therefore, a common form of parental discipline toward their children.

Several factors and conditions have been associated with parental violence, including parent characteristics (i.e., parents' own experience of child maltreatment, age and educational level, cognitive ability, and personality), child characteristics (i.e., age and sex), and sociodemographic conditions (i.e., household income, number of children in the household) [42–44]. Low-income and economic hardship strain parents' mental health, increase the likelihood of family conflict, and reduce interaction among family members in a responsive and nurturing manner, which predict poor child developmental outcomes [45–47].

Also, parental beliefs and cultural acceptance that corporal punishment is a way to raise and educate their children to contribute to these forms of discipline have not been yet abandoned. Even in wealthy and considered highly developed societies, such as Switzerland, it was estimated that 54.4% of children aged 1–14 suffered forms of corporal punishment at home [48]. In the United States, corporal punishment remains a legal and well-accepted form of disciplining children, with prevalence studies reporting 64–95% of parents use spanking between the ages of 2 and 3 [49]. Worldwide, one in four adults reports having been physically abused as a child by their parents or other caregivers [12], three-quarters of world children aged 2 to 4 are regularly victims of violent discipline by their parents or other caregivers [50], and around six in 10 children aged 2–14 are frequently punished physically [51]. However, a growing number of countries are passing laws prohibiting its use at home. A study conducted in the scope of a Portuguese population-based cohort (the Generation XXI) showed a high prevalence of physical violent discipline [52]. In this study, the parent-child Conflict Tactics Scale (CTSPC) was administered to 4175 children by trained interviewers to report parents' disciplinary practices. This instrument includes 23 items that allow us to measure three different forms of lifetime parental disciplinary acts: (1) non-violent discipline, characterized by positive practices widely used as alternatives to corporal punishment; (2) psychological aggression, which includes verbal and symbolic acts to cause psychological pain or fear to the child; and (3) physical assault, which comprises the use of corporal punishment that may include acts of physical abuse. An interviewer shows the child a picture card and reads a description, such as "This girl's father hits her with a belt when she does something wrong. When you do something wrong, does your father hit you with a belt?" If the response is yes, the interviewer shows a second card with the response categories in the form of stacked circles that the child could point to. Answers to the child-report form items were rated using a 5-point Likert-type scale, ranging from "Never" to "Always," with higher scores indicating a higher occurrence of the parental disciplinary act. Child-reported discipline practices used by parents were recoded as "never" if the child did not report any act of parental violent discipline, as "sometimes" if the child reported that the tactic occurred "once" or "sometimes" and as "frequently" if the child reported its occurrence as "frequently" and "always."

Table 1 shows the frequency of physical violence reported by the children. These results show us the high frequency of corporal punishment as a tactic of parental discipline. In Portugal, although a Law introduced in 2007 has amended the Portuguese Penal Code to prohibit all forms of corporal punishment of children, including by parents [53], physical discipline is still observed.

Also, the social environment in which a child is born and raised affects the nature and quality of social relations and interactions, which, in turn, impacts growth, development, and future achievements. In literature, it has been described that a warm and sensitive parenting style contributes to a child's positive social behavior and supportive peer relationships [54]. In contrast, unstable, neglectful, or abusive families are associated with episodes of aggressiveness, and impulsivity in the children, impairing their development of tactics to solve a conflict with peers [55], and increasing the risk of violent, aggressive, and bullying behaviors in settings, such as school, that is, outside home environments [56].

Results from the children followed by the cohort Generation XXI showed an increased likelihood of involvement as a bully in children from families with a history of household criminality, that witness parental violence and victims of physical

		n (%)
Corporal punishment	Never	671 (16.1)
	Sometimes	867 (20.8)
	Frequently	2637 (63.1)
Severe physical assault	Never	3605 (86.3)
	Sometimes	401 (9.6)
	Frequently	169 (4.1)
Very severe physical assault	Never	4056 (97.1)
	Sometimes	95 (2.3)
	Frequently	24 (0.6)

Table 1.
Prevalence of parental physical violence (assessed with the Parent-Child Conflict Tactics Scale) in a sample of 7-year-old children from Generation XXI, a birth cohort from Porto, Portugal (N = 4175).

violence [57]. These findings suggest that exposure to household dysfunction might impact children's emotional and behavioral development. Thus, being exposed to or witnessing other forms of victimization at home might increase their susceptibility to being involved in bullying [58], as children might see it as an acceptable way to manage interpersonal conflicts.

2.3 Peer violence

Children are entitled and must be provided with a safe, nurturing, and inclusive environment where they can grow, learn, thrive, and succeed, achieving their full potential as students and citizens [59]. Communities devote their confidence and expect that schools are the providers of such non-violent environments. However, students all over the world see their ability to fully benefit from educational opportunities endangered by the presence or threat of violence at school, exerted mainly by their peers.

Violence among school-age children and adolescents is a worldwide problem, with negative impact and consequences for the physical and psychological health of those involved, and also, increased risk of behavioral and social problems [12]. Violence at school has also other consequences, such as lower rates of attendance, contributes to lower academic results, and leads to higher drop-out rates [50].

The most traditional forms of peer violence occurring in the educational context comprise bullying, cyberbullying, and physical fighting.

Bullying is an intentional aggressive and negative behavior, repeated over time, that involves a power imbalance favoring the aggressor, with victims having no means to defend themselves [60]. The most common forms of bullying behaviors among adolescents are name-calling, teasing, making threats, spreading rumors, taking of personal belongings, and rejection by excluding someone from a group on purpose [61]. Most of the bullying situations tend to start in school, and sometimes they are not taken as seriously but, instead, as a normal interaction between peers [62]. Children or adolescents involved in bullying can dress the role of victims when the child suffers from bullying but is not an aggressor; as bullies, when the involvement is sole as the aggressor, but not as a victim; and as bully-victim when the child is involved as both victim and aggressor simultaneously.

Estimates of bullying prevalence vary greatly across surveys. A survey conducted by the Health Behavior in School-Aged Children (HBSC) study, in 42 countries and regions across the World Health Organization (WHO) European Region and North America, showed that between 3 and 35% of young people reported involvement in bullying during the past 2 months [63]. According to the WHO European Health Information Gateway from 2017, 11% of girls and 17% of boys aged 11 years old, and 14% of girls and 16% of boys aged 13 have reported being victims of bullying at least twice in the previous 2 months [64].

In a study conducted in the scope of a Portuguese population-based cohort (the Generation XXI) the bullying behavior was assessed through the Bully Scale Survey developed by the Centers for Disease Control and Prevention (CDC) [65]. This scale collects information on the experience of bullying as a victim (11 items) and as a bully (11 items). At the age of 10 years, for each item, the child was asked to indicate the frequency of bullying involvement, choosing between five options—"never," "rarely," "sometimes," "often," and "always." As bullying is a repeated behavior, the child was categorized as a victim, when reporting the occurrence of at least one of the items as "often" or "always" in the victimization scale, but answered "never," "rarely," or "sometimes" in the aggression scale; the child was classified as a "bully" when answered "often" or "always" in the aggression scale, but answered "never," "rarely," or "sometimes" in the victimization scale; finally, the child was categorized as "bully-victim" when reported to be involved both as a victim and as an aggressor simultaneously.

Figure 1 shows results from 5338 participants of Generation XXI. Overall, near 20% of children aged 10 years reported to have been involved in bullying; involvement as only the victim was reported by 14.4% of participants, involvement as only-bully by 1.4%, and involvement as both bully and victim by 3.9%. Boys were more frequently involved in bullying than girls (16.6% versus 12.0% as victims; 2.0% versus 0.7% as bullies; and 5.5% versus 2.3% as bully-victims) [57].

In our society, gender constitutes a structure of social practice that establishes relations of power, attitudes, and hierarchies among people, groups, and institutions [66], and this is reflected in the interaction between children, and consequently in bullying behaviors. Research suggests that boys are more prone to be victims and aggressors of bullying, especially in its physical expression [63, 67], while girls are more likely to engage in situations of indirect bullying, such as teasing or gossiping [62, 67, 68].

With the democratization of the use of new technologies and social media, a new form of peer violence has emerged, cyberbullying, that uses that platform as the scenario for the perpetration of aggressive behaviors [69]. Cyberbullying is the act of sending, posting, or sharing negative, harmful, false, or mean content about someone else through SMS, MMS, and apps, or online in social media, forums, or gaming where people can view, participate in, or share content. It aims to share personal or private information about someone else to cause embarrassment or humiliation. Some cyberbullying crosses the line into unlawful or criminal behavior [70].

However, as for bullying, the prevalence of cyberbullying estimates varies greatly across surveys. A previous scoping review described the prevalence of lifetime cybervictimization as ranging between 4.9 and 65.0%, prevalence of aggression ranging between 1.2 and 44.1%, and prevalence of being involved as victim and aggressor simultaneously ranging from 5.0 to 64.3% [71]. It is known that the attacks cause greater insecurity in the victim, as there are no places or moments to hide

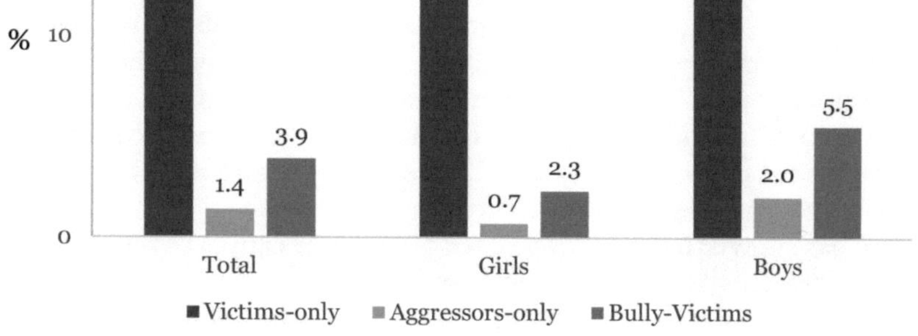

Figure 1.
Prevalence of bullying by sex according to the type of involvement assessed (victimization, aggression, and victimization and aggression simultaneously) among 10-year-old children.

since aggressors can reach them almost everywhere [72]. In addition, due to how the violence is carried out, it can be observed by numerous bystanders for an indefinite number of times, which makes the potential damage even greater than that of traditional harassment [72]. Due to the potential of widespread accessibility of victims and an infinite audience by using communication technologies [73], cyberbullying is another important source of stress. Thus, we should also be monitoring the use of technologies as a common form of violence at these ages.

Physical fighting has been measured as a form of violence strongly related to violence in a community. This form of violence is of easy assessment and considered one of the main causes of child morbidity and mortality, accounting for one of the leading causes of death among adolescents aged 15 or over in Europe and America [74]. Physical fighting is defined as the use of an intentional force against others, with potentially serious consequences and injuries or death [75].

Particularly, there is a significant association between physical fighting involvement and other violent behaviors, such as carrying weapons and greater involvement in risk behaviors, being often associated with substance misuse, such as alcohol and drug use [75–78], as well as media violence exposure [79, 80]. Studies examining the association between both the quantity and quality of sleep and aggression behavior among male adolescents showed that hostility was associated with both reduced quantity [81] and quality of sleep [82].

3. Consequences of violence for health in childhood and adolescence

Violence can have different impacts and effects on the health of children and adolescents. Literature shows that exposure to stressful and traumatic experiences during sensitive periods of neurological and cognitive development in childhood may have lasting implications for physical, emotional, and mental health [12, 83] being a significant early determinant of disease onset and all-cause premature mortality [84–86].

The physical impacts of violence episodes are the most easily observable and recognizable and may include mild or serious wounds, bruises, fractures. However, we cannot discard that some violence experiences are not so visible but have a significant impact on children's future health and well-being.

Regarding parental violence, parental and cultural beliefs that corporal punishment is an acceptable way to discipline and educate children, contribute to these forms of discipline not being yet abandoned. However, corporal punishment is responsible for thousands of deaths during childhood each year and regarding its survivors, it has been associated with health problems in childhood and later in life [87]. Given the stigmatizing nature of violence, and its occurrence in a place where the child is supposed to be safe, mostly perpetrated by the ones that should be the main protectors of the child by providing them with a healthy and safe environment, over-reporting is not common, and it is expected that prevalence estimates tend to underestimate the true magnitude of interpersonal violence.

Literature has shown that any experience of violence causes psychological distress and long-term mental ill-health [88]. Exposure to household conflicts poses a significant threat to children's ability to process and regulate emotions, and it may result in uncontrolled or overcontrolled emotional reactions, contributing to both internalizing and externalizing behaviors [89]. Also, victims of corporal punishment both at home and at school are more likely to become passive and excessively cautious and to a fear-free expression of their ideas and feelings. Children who suffer physical punishment are less likely than other children to internalize moral values, to be altruistic, empathic, or to exercise moral judgment of any kind. Also, being a victim of both physical and psychological abuse increases the risk of depression, posttraumatic stress disorder (PTSD), and anxiety [90, 91].

The involvement in physical fights and bullying victimization is related to somatic symptoms and disturbances, reflecting the emotional effects of aggression. Adolescents involved in physical fights are more likely to present negative health outcomes, such as sleep problems, appetite suppression, and headaches [92, 93]. Similarly, in victims of bullying the most common stress-related symptoms include sleep disorders [94], gastrointestinal complaints, headaches, chronic pain [62, 95], and also bedwetting and tummy ache [96].

Additionally, a girl victim of bullying is at higher risk of suicidal ideation, feeling more nervous or stressed and angry than a boy [97]. One possible explanation is the fact that girls seem to externalize their emotions better and disclose their depressive feelings more easily than boys [62, 98, 99]. Results from a study conducted with adolescents showed that those involved in bullying were more likely to present negative well-being-related feelings, including feeling "nervous or stressed," "angry," "sad and desperate," and also "suicidal ideation." Suicidal ideation was strongly associated with being involved in bullying as bully-victim, in girls (OR = 8.34; 95% CI: 5.03; 3.82) and in boys (OR = 8.05; 95% CI: 4.24; 15.28) [67].

The link between violence and health may be explained by the biology of social adversity. Therefore, the exposure to violence during childhood may result in early life stress that has the potential to alter physiological systems, thus accounting for a more immediate effect of these exposures, including all the effects that occurred during childhood and adolescence, before adulthood, but that may not necessarily lead to disease. Although the mechanisms explaining the involvement in the biological embodiment of violence are poorly understood in early ages, accumulating evidence suggests that adversity may become programmed molecularly, leaving behind biological memories that can persistently translate into an increased susceptibility to disease later in life [100–102].

Inflammation, for instance, may be one of the potential mechanisms explaining the link between trauma and health outcomes. Longitudinal studies showed that elevated markers of inflammation, namely C-reactive protein (CRP) levels were observed in adults who experienced childhood adversity, such as parental separation [103], child maltreatment [104], and low socioeconomic status [105]. CRP is an acute-phase protein of hepatic origin whose circulating concentrations rise in response to inflammation. In hospital settings, it can be used to determine the risk of developing coronary artery disease. Although the health effects of violence are well documented in adults, more and more literature has been showing that these alterations start at very early ages. A systematic review aimed to summarize evidence reporting epigenetic and/or neuro-immuno-endocrine embedding of adverse childhood experiences, including violence and episodes of bullying, in children, with a particular focus on the short-term biological effect of those events [106]. The authors observed that the associations reported across studies followed the hypothesis that exposure to adversity is associated with increased biological alterations already at early ages, which may increase the risk of later health outcomes [106].

Empirical data from a birth cohort from Portugal, Generation XXI, showed that at the age of 7 years, children who reported more severe violence perpetrated by their parents presented significantly higher levels of hs-CRP [52]. Higher hs-CRP levels were observed among children reporting extreme violence, including "grab the children by the neck and choke them" or "burn the children or scald them on purpose" [52].

This is supporting evidence that adversity appears to get "under the skin" and induce physiological changes. Although little is known if these alterations in biological markers after experiencing abuse at early ages may be reversed, these results seem to support evidence for biological imprinting and short-term physiological effect of violence that might be strongly associated with later development of disease.

Due to some specificities regarding the type of involvement, bullying might have a different biological impact or health consequences depending on the involvement as a victim, aggressor, or both simultaneously. While evidence has shown that being bullied predicted higher increases in CRP levels, bullying others predicted lower increases in CRP compared with those uninvolved in bullying [107]. A systematic review [106] described other health consequences that were observed, such as higher DNA methylation, shorter telomere length [108], and lower cortisol levels among victims of bullying [109]. However, further investigation is needed to explore the impact of children's type of involvement in bullying on different biological markers.

In conclusion, literature shows that violence and toxic stress induce physiological changes already in childhood and put children at increased risk for developing several diseases in adulthood, negatively impacting their quality of life and setting them in a less advantageous position [110, 111] from the early life onwards. Exposure to psychosocial stressors leads to continuous dysregulation of physiological responses resulting in the wear and tear on the body, an allostatic load with detrimental long-term health consequences [112].

4. Overcoming and thriving adversity: the resilience framework

Despite growing up and living in contexts of violence, not all children will develop the illness. Some of them even present indicators of healthy development, demonstrating to be resilient to such a disadvantaged environment [113]. The impact of social disadvantage in childhood and allostatic load in later life can be modified by individuals' psychosocial resilience [112].

Resilience is the individuals' capacity for overcoming the negative effects of risk exposure, coping successfully with adverse experiences as well as avoiding the negative trajectories associated with risk. This process is influenced by biological, psychological, social, and contextual factors [114]. The most consistent protective factors associated with resilience in children exposed to violence recognized by the literature are supportive parent-child relationships at a family level and self-regulation at an individual level [113].

Examining what differentiates children who demonstrate resilience from those who develop illness and assessing their ability to cope with unfavorable events is essential for informing interventions aiming to improve coping skills and competences promoting healthy trajectories [110, 115, 116]. The identification of the multidimensional processes underlying successful adaptation under adverse conditions allows the design and implementation of successful interventions for the most vulnerable children.

Resiliency Theory focuses on strengths rather than deficits, giving attention to assets (i.e., individual protective factors, such as social skills, coping skills, healthy beliefs, and self-efficacy) and resources (i.e., social and environmental context strengthening individuals facing the risk) which help children to be healthy adults and to have a good quality of life [114, 117, 118]. Studies on Resiliency Theory use three models of resilience—the compensatory, protective, and challenge models—to explain the processes by which promotive factors positively influence the adversity trajectories [114]. The compensatory model defends the idea of a promotive factor acting in an opposite direction of a risk factor on an outcome. The protective factor model highlights the moderating effect of assets and resources on the relationships between a risk factor and a negative outcome. The challenge model suggests that the exposure to moderate levels of a risk factor is associated with less negative, or even positive, outcomes, while low levels and high levels of a risk factor are associated with negative outcomes [114].

Recent studies on the impact of advantageous childhood experiences on adult health have been using the compensatory model of Resiliency Theory, defending that positive childhood experiences will have a direct influence on an outcome [117], counteracting the negative effects of adverse events [118]. The cumulative number of childhood positive experiences leading to resilience and better lifelong health are considered as counter-ACES, including positive parenting, school involvement, meaningful beliefs, and positive and close relationships with family, friends, and other adults [117, 119].

Positive and advantageous childhood experiences and supportive relationships may improve future social experiences and healthy relationships, protecting children against poor health and promoting well-being throughout life [119, 120]. To reduce health problems and improve the quality of life of vulnerable populations, it may be more important to increase counter-ACEs than decrease ACEs. Public health programs focusing on counter-ACEs are able to help families and communities to surround vulnerable children with counter-ACEs, such as parent-child attachment or household routines, helping to neutralize the negative effect of ACEs on children's health and well-being [120].

Studying childhood maltreatment with a resiliency framework can be particularly important due to the harmful and long-term effects of violence in childhood. This framework allows us to analyze the positive and negative trajectories of children who experienced violence, to understand how maltreated and neglected children overcome the adverse experiences, and to explore the processes, moderators, and mechanisms that facilitate a positive adaptation to violence [121].

Previous studies highlight the important role of families, schools, and peers as well as of individuals' self-regulation in promoting a positive developmental trajectory in children exposed to violence [113]. The existence of a supportive and stable carer is one of the most important protective factors associated with positive outcomes in this population [121]. Therefore, health promotion strategies directed to children living in violent contexts should be focused on strengthening supportive relationships across ecological contexts, including families, schools, and communities, and on the development of school-based programs aiming at developing children's self-regulatory capacities [113].

In conclusion, there is a need to deepen the knowledge on childhood resilience to inform the design and development of public health intervention strategies and policies to relieve the impact of violence suffered by individuals during their developmental years, allowing them to achieve good health and quality of life. These strategies will give children living in adverse environments hope and tools to change their negative path, tackling costly social and health inequities. Building resilience in early childhood offers an opportunity to improve the quality of life of the next generation, enhance productivity, and reduce healthcare costs [122].

5. Conclusions

Growing up in a context of violence mostly perpetrated by the ones that should be the main protectors of the child by providing them with a healthy and safe environment may trigger a cascade of psychosocial vulnerabilities. The child may be vulnerable to being exposed to violence at home and then at school, and these experiences can be manifested in different ways. Regardless of the type of exposure to violence, it has a serious impact on child health and development. Although assessing violence experiences in cohort studies may be challenging, it is very relevant to include these questions in the cohort assessments. First, it is a human rights question; second, it impacts the child's development and well-being; and third, it will impact long-term health. A longitudinal perspective will contribute to understanding the intersection of different violent experiences and their contribution to the production of health inequalities. In addition, we can explore the resilience factors in a life-course perspective, which will help to inform the design and development of interventions enhancing existing skills, encouraging healthy adjustment trajectories, and nurturing resilient adaptation.

Acknowledgements

The authors would like to acknowledge the vision of Professor Henrique Barros for always considering violence as a relevant topic for public health and including measures of violence in the cohort assessments.

Support for the completion of this work was provided by the European Regional Development Fund (ERDF) through the Operational Programme Competitiveness and Internationalization and national funding from the Foundation for Science and Technology (FCT), Portuguese Ministry of Science, Technology and Higher Education through the financing of the project "HIneC: When do health inequalities start? Understanding the impact of childhood social adversity on health trajectories from birth to early adolescence" (POCI-01-0145-FEDER-029567; PTDC/SAU-PUB/29567/2017), the Epidemiology Research Unit—Instituto de Saúde Pública da Universidade do Porto (EPIUnit) (UIDB/04750/2020), the Associate Laboratory ITR (LA/P/0064/2020), and the individual researcher contract to SF (CEECIND/01516/2017).

Conflict of interest

The authors declare no conflict of interest.

DOI: http://dx.doi.org/10.5772/intechopen.102581

Author details

Sílvia Fraga*, Mariana Amorim and Sara Soares
Institute of Public Health, University of Porto, Porto, Portugal

*Address all correspondence to: silvia.fraga@ispup.up.pt

References

[1] Brady SS. Lifetime community violence exposure and health risk behavior among young adults in college. The Journal of Adolescent Health. 2006; **39**(4):610-613

[2] Cairney J, Krause N. Negative life events and age-related decline in mastery: Are older adults more vulnerable to the control-eroding effect of stress? The Journals of Gerontology. Series B, Psychological Sciences and Social Sciences. 2008;**63**(3):S162-S170

[3] Campbell J, Jones AS, Dienemann J, Kub J, Schollenberger J, O'Campo P, et al. Intimate partner violence and physical health consequences. Archives of Internal Medicine. 2002;**162**(10):1157-1163

[4] Heise L, Ellsberg M, Gottmoeller M. A global overview of gender-based violence. International Journal of Gynecology and Obstetrics. 2002; **78**(S1):S5-S14

[5] Elder GH. The life course as developmental theory. Child Development. 1998;**69**(1):1-12

[6] Macmillan R. Violence and the life course: The consequences of victimization for personal and social development. Annual Review of Sociology. 2001;**27**(1):1-22

[7] Robins LNRM. Straight and Devious Pathways from Childhood to Adulthood. Cambridge, New York: Cambridge University Press; 1990

[8] Fraga S. Methodological and ethical challenges in violence research. Porto Biomedical Journal. 2016;**1**(2):77-80

[9] Kinard EM. Ethical issues in research with abused children. Child Abuse and Neglect. 1985;**9**(3):301-311

[10] Kinard EM. Methodological issues and practical problems in conducting research on maltreated children. Child Abuse and Neglect. 1994;**18**(8):645-656

[11] Johnston JR, Lee S, Olesen NW, Walters MG. Allegations and substantiations of abuse in custody-disputing families. Family Court Review. 2005;**43**(2):283-294

[12] World Health Organization. Global Status Report on Violence Prevention. Geneve: World Health Organization; 2014

[13] Hillis S, Mercy J, Amobi A, Kress H. Global prevalence of past-year violence against children: A systematic review and minimum estimates. Pediatrics. 2016;**137**(3):e20154079

[14] Bowers A, Strelitz J, Allen J, Donkin A. An Equal Start: Improving outcomes in Children's Centres, the Evidence Review. London: University College London; 2012

[15] Pillas D, Marmot M, Naicker K, Goldblatt P, Morrison J, Pikhart H. Social inequalities in early childhood health and development: A European-wide systematic review. Pediatric Research. 2014;**76**(5):418-424

[16] Commission on Social Determinants of Health. Closing the Gap in a Generation. Geneva: World Health Organization; 2008

[17] Burman M, Öhman A, editors. Challenging gender and violence: Positions and discourses in Swedish and international contexts. Women's Studies International Forum. 2014;**46**:81-82

[18] Talge NM, Neal C, Glover V. Antenatal maternal stress and long-term

effects on child neurodevelopment: How and why? Journal of Child Psychology and Psychiatry. 2007;**48**(3-4):245-261

[19] Rosen D, Seng JS, Tolman RM, Mallinger G. Intimate partner violence, depression, and posttraumatic stress disorder as additional predictors of low birth weight infants among low-income mothers. Journal of Interpersonal Violence. 2007;**22**(10):1305-1314

[20] Sarkar NN. The impact of intimate partner violence on women's reproductive health and pregnancy outcome. Journal of Obstetrics and Gynaecology. 2008;**28**(3):266-271

[21] Rodrigues T, Rocha L, Barros H. Physical abuse during pregnancy and preterm delivery. American Journal of Obstetrics and Gynecology. 2008;**198**(2):171.e1-171.e6

[22] Han A, Stewart DE. Maternal and fetal outcomes of intimate partner violence associated with pregnancy in the Latin American and Caribbean region. International Journal of Gynaecology and Obstetrics. 2014;**124**(1):6-11

[23] Janssen PA, Holt VL, Sugg NK, Emanuel I, Critchlow CM, Henderson AD. Intimate partner violence and adverse pregnancy outcomes: A population-based study. American Journal of Obstetrics and Gynecology. 2003;**188**(5):1341-1347

[24] Donovan BM, Spracklen CN, Schweizer ML, Ryckman KK, Saftlas AF. Intimatepartnerviolenceduringpregnancy and the risk for adverse infant outcomes: A systematic review and meta-analysis. BJOG: An International Journal of Obstetrics and Gynaecology. 2016;**123**(8):1289-1299

[25] Cnattingius S. The epidemiology of smoking during pregnancy: Smoking prevalence, maternal characteristics, and pregnancy outcomes. Nicotine and Tobacco Research. 2004;**6**(Suppl. 2): S125-S140

[26] Dube SR, Miller JW, Brown DW, Giles WH, Felitti VJ, Dong M, et al. Adverse childhood experiences and the association with ever using alcohol and initiating alcohol use during adolescence. Journal of Adolescent Health. 2006;**38**(4):444.e1-444.10

[27] Lester BM, Tronick EZ, LaGasse L, Seifer R, Bauer CR, Shankaran S, et al. The maternal lifestyle study: Effects of substance exposure during pregnancy on neurodevelopmental outcome in 1-month-old infants. Pediatrics. 2002;**110**(6):1182-1192

[28] Williamson DF, Thompson TJ, Anda RF, Dietz WH, Felitti V. Body weight and obesity in adults and self-reported abuse in childhood. International Journal of Obesity and Related Metabolic Disorders. 2002;**26**(8):1075-1082

[29] Charil A, Laplante DP, Vaillancourt C, King S. Prenatal stress and brain development. Brain Research Reviews. 2010;**65**(1):56-79

[30] Mehler MF, Purpura DP. Autism, fever, epigenetics and the locus coeruleus. Brain Research Reviews. 2009;**59**(2):388-392

[31] Conradt E, Lester BM, Appleton AA, Armstrong DA, Marsit CJ. The roles of DNA methylation of NR3C1 and 11β-HSD2 and exposure to maternal mood disorder in utero on newborn neurobehavior. Epigenetics. 2013; **8**(12):1321-1329

[32] Kinney DK, Miller AM, Crowley DJ, Huang E, Gerber E. Autism prevalence following prenatal exposure to

hurricanes and tropical storms in Louisiana. Journal of Autism and Developmental Disorders. 2008; **38**(3):481-488

[33] Radtke KM, Ruf M, Gunter HM, Dohrmann K, Schauer M, Meyer A, et al. Transgenerational impact of intimate partner violence on methylation in the promoter of the glucocorticoid receptor. Translational Psychiatry. 2011;**1**(7):e21-e21

[34] Dietert RR, Dietert JM. Potential for early-life immune insult including developmental immunotoxicity in autism and autism spectrum disorders: Focus on critical windows of immune vulnerability. Journal of Toxicology and Environmental Health. Part B, Critical Reviews. 2008;**11**(8):660-680

[35] Roberts AL, Lyall K, Rich-Edwards JW, Ascherio A, Weisskopf MG. Maternal exposure to intimate partner abuse before birth is associated with autism spectrum disorder in offspring. Autism. 2016;**20**(1):26-36

[36] Grizenko N, Fortier M-E, Zadorozny C, Thakur G, Schmitz N, Duval R. Maternal stress during pregnancy, ADHD symptomatology in children and genotype: Gene-environment interaction. Journal of the Canadian Academy of Child and Adolescent Psychiatry. 2012;**21**:9-15

[37] Laplante DP, Barr RG, Brunet A, Galbaud du Fort G, Meaney ML, Saucier JF, et al. Stress during pregnancy affects general intellectual and language functioning in human toddlers. Pediatric Research. 2004;**56**(3):400-410

[38] Davis EP, Sandman CA. The timing of prenatal exposure to maternal cortisol and psychosocial stress is associated with human infant cognitive development. Child Development. 2010;**81**(1):131-148

[39] Bogat GA, DeJonghe E, Levendosky AA, Davidson WS, von Eye A. Trauma symptoms among infants exposed to intimate partner violence. Child Abuse and Neglect. 2006;**30**(2):109-125

[40] Kempe CH, Silverman FN, Steele BF, Droegemueller W, Silver HK. The battered-child syndrome. Journal of the American Medical Association. 1962;**181**(1):17-24

[41] World Health Organization. Preventing child maltreatment: A Guide to Taking Action and Generating Evidence/World Health Organization and International Society for Prevention of Child Abuse and Neglect. Geneva: World Health Organization; 2006

[42] Creavey KL, Gatzke-Kopp LM, Fosco GM. Differential effects of family stress exposure and harsh parental discipline on child social competence. Journal of Child and Family Studies. 2018;**27**(2):483-493

[43] Friedson M. Authoritarian parenting attitudes and social origin: The multigenerational relationship of socioeconomic position to childrearing values. Child Abuse and Neglect. 2016;**51**:263-275

[44] Yunus KRM, Dahlan NA. Child-rearing practices and socio-economic status: Possible implications for children's educational outcomes. Procedia—Social and Behavioral Sciences. 2013;**90**:251-259

[45] Chen E, Miller GE. Socioeconomic status and health: Mediating and moderating factors. Annual Review of Clinical Psychology. 2013;**9**:723-749

[46] Gülseven Z, Kumru A, Carlo G, Palermo F, Selçuk B, Sayıl M. The mediational roles of harsh and responsive parenting in the longitudinal relations between socioeconomic

status and Turkish children's emotional development. International Journal of Behavioral Development. 2018;**42**(6):563-573

[47] Roubinov DS, Boyce WT. Parenting and SES: Relative values or enduring principles? Current Opinion in Psychology. 2017;**15**:162-167

[48] UNICEF. Know Violence in Childhood. Ending Violence in Childhood. 2017

[49] Straus MA. Prevalence, societal causes, and trends in corporal punishment by parents in world perspective. Law and Contemporary Problems. 2010;**73**(2):1-30

[50] United Nations Children's Fund. A Familiar Face: Violence in the lives of children and adolescents. New York: UNICEF; 2017

[51] UNICEF. Hidden in Plain Sight: A Statistical Analysis of Violence against Children. 2014. Available from: https://www.unicef.org/publications/index_74865.html

[52] Fraga S, Soares S, Santos AC, Barros H. Parents' use of extreme physical violence is associated with elevated high-sensitivity C-reactive protein in children. Journal of Affective Disorders. 2021;**282**:454-457

[53] Decreto-Lei nº. 48/95 - Violência doméstica. 2007

[54] Helsen M, Vollebergh W, Meeus W. Social support from parents and friends and emotional problems in adolescence. Journal of youth and adolescence. 2000;**29**(3):319-335

[55] Van der Kolk BA. Developmental. Psychiatric Annals. 2005;**35**(5):401

[56] Hong JS, Espelage DL. A review of research on bullying and peer victimization in school: An ecological system analysis. Aggression and Violent Behavior. 2012;**17**(4):311-322

[57] Fraga S, Soares S, Peres FS, Barros H. Household dysfunction is associated with bullying behavior in 10-year-old children: Do socioeconomic circumstances matter? Journal of Interpersonal Violence. 2021;**0**(0):08862605211006352

[58] Lereya ST, Copeland WE, Costello EJ, Wolke D. Adult mental health consequences of peer bullying and maltreatment in childhood: Two cohorts in two countries. The Lancet Psychiatry. 2015;**2**(6):524-531

[59] United Nations. SDG-Education. 2030 Steering Committee. 2015. Available from: https://sustainabledevelopment.un.org/index.php?page=view&type=30022&nr=100&menu=3170

[60] Olweus D. Bullying at school: What we know and what we can do. Psychology in the Schools. 1993;**40**(6):699-700

[61] Smith PK, Cowie H, Olafsson RF, Liefooghe AP, Almeida A, Araki H, et al. Definitions of bullying: A comparison of terms used, and age and gender differences, in a fourteen-country international comparison. Child Development. 2002;**73**(4):1119-1133

[62] National Academies of Sciences, Engineering and Medicine. Preventing Bullying Through Science, Policy, and Practice. Washington, DC: The National Academies Press; 2016

[63] Craig WM, Harel Y. Bullying, physical fighting and victimization. Young People's Health in Context: International Report from the HBSC. 2001;**2**:133-144

[64] World Health Organization. Child and Adolescent Health. 2017.

Available from: https://www.who.int/news-room/fact-sheets/detail/adolescents-health-risks-and-solutions

[65] Hamburger ME, Basile KC, Vivolo AM. Measuring Bullying Victimization, Perpetration, and Bystander Experiences; A Compendium of Assessment Tools. National Center for Injury Prevention and Control (US), Division of Violence Prevention. 2011

[66] Steinfeldt JA, Vaughan EL, LaFollette JR, Steinfeldt MC. Bullying among adolescent football players: Role of masculinity and moral atmosphere. Psychology of Men and Masculinity. 2012;**13**(4):340-353

[67] Silva-Rocha N, Soares S, Brochado S, Fraga S. Bullying involvement, family background, school life, and well-being feelings among adolescents. Journal of Public Health. 2020;**28**(5):481-489

[68] Finkelhor D, Shattuck A, Turner H, Hamby S. A revised inventory of adverse childhood experiences. Child Abuse and Neglect. 2015;**48**:13-21

[69] Aboujaoude E, Savage MW, Starcevic V, Salame WO. Cyberbullying: Review of an old problem gone viral. Journal of Adolescent Health. 2015;**57**(1):10-18

[70] U.S. Department of Health and Human Services. What Is Cyberbullying Washington: StopBullying.gov. 2017. Available from: https://www.stopbullying.gov/cyberbullying/what-is-it

[71] Brochado S, Fraga S, Soares S, Ramos E, Barros H. Cyberbullying among adolescents: The influence of different modes of inquiry. Journal of Interpersonal Violence. 2017;**36**(3-4):1933-1950

[72] Smith PK, Mahdavi J, Carvalho M, Fisher S, Russell S, Tippett N. Cyberbullying: Its nature and impact in secondary school pupils. Journal of Child Psychology and Psychiatry. 2008;**49**(4):376-385

[73] Shariff S, Hoff DL. Cyber bullying: Clarifying Legal Boundaries for School Supervision in Cyberspace. 2016

[74] Mokdad AH, Forouzanfar MH, Daoud F, Mokdad AA, El Bcheraoui C, Moradi-Lakeh M, et al. Global burden of diseases, injuries, and risk factors for young people's health during 1990-2013: A systematic analysis for the global burden of disease study 2013. Lancet. 2016;**387**(10036):2383-2401

[75] Pickett W, Molcho M, Elgar FJ, Brooks F, de Looze M, Rathmann K, et al. Trends and socioeconomic correlates of adolescent physical fighting in 30 countries. Pediatrics. 2013;**131**(1):e18-e26

[76] Fraga S, Ramos E, Dias S, Barros H. Physical fighting among school-going Portuguese adolescents: Social and behavioural correlates. Preventive Medicine. 2011;**52**(5):401-404

[77] Rudatsikira E, Muula AS, Siziya S. Prevalence and correlates of physical fighting among school-going adolescents in Santiago, Chile. Brazilian Journal of Psychiatry. 2008;**30**(3):197-202

[78] Swahn MH, Bossarte RM, Palmier JB, Yao H, Van Dulmen MHM. Psychosocial characteristics associated with frequent physical fighting: Findings from the 2009 National Youth Risk Behavior Survey. Injury Prevention. 2013;**19**(2):143-146

[79] Coker TR, Elliott MN, Schwebel DC, Windle M, Toomey SL, Tortolero SR, et al. Media violence exposure and physical aggression in fifth-grade children. Academic Pediatrics. 2015;**15**(1):82-88

[80] Demissie Z, Lowry R, Eaton DK, Hertz MF, Lee SM. Associations of school violence with physical activity among U.S. high school students. Journal of Physical Activity and Health. 2014;**11**(4):705-711

[81] Soares S, Araújo J, Ramos E, Fraga S. Sleep duration and physical fighting involvement in late adolescence. Journal of Public Health. 2019;**27**(3):341-348

[82] Ireland JL, Culpin V. The relationship between sleeping problems and aggression, anger, and impulsivity in a population of juvenile and young offenders. Journal of Adolescent Health. 2006;**38**(6):649-655

[83] Anda RF, Felitti VJ, Bremner JD, Walker JD, Whitfield C, Perry BD, et al. The enduring effects of abuse and related adverse experiences in childhood. A convergence of evidence from neurobiology and epidemiology. European Archives of Psychiatry and Clinical Neuroscience. 2006;**256**(3):174-186

[84] Felitti VJ, Anda RF, Nordenberg D, Williamson DF, Spitz AM, Edwards V, et al. Relationship of childhood abuse and household dysfunction to many of the leading causes of death in adults. The Adverse Childhood Experiences (ACE) Study. American Journal of Preventive Medicine. 1998;**14**(4):245-258

[85] Kelly-Irving M, Mabile L, Grosclaude P, Lang T, Delpierre C. The embodiment of adverse childhood experiences and cancer development: Potential biological mechanisms and pathways across the life course. International journal of public health. 2012;**58**(1):3-11

[86] Miller GE, Chen E, Parker KJ. Psychological stress in childhood and susceptibility to the chronic diseases of aging: Moving toward a model of behavioral and biological mechanisms. Psychological Bulletin. 2011;**137**(6):959-997

[87] World Health Organization. Chapter 3: Child Abuse and Neglect by Parents and other Caregivers. Geneva: World Health Organization; 2002

[88] Ferrara P, Franceschini G, Villani A, Corsello G. Physical, psychological and social impact of school violence on children. Italian Journal of Pediatrics. 2019;**45**(1):76

[89] Zarling AL, Taber-Thomas S, Murray A, Knuston JF, Lawrence E, Valles N-L, et al. Internalizing and externalizing symptoms in young children exposed to intimate partner violence: Examining intervening processes. Journal of Family Psychology. 2013;**27**(6):945

[90] Dillon G, Hussain R, Loxton D, Rahman S. Mental and physical health and intimate partner violence against women: A review of the literature. International Journal of Family Medicine. 2013;**2013**:313909

[91] Lawrence E, Orengo-Aguayo R, Langer A, Brock R. The impact and consequences of partner abuse on partners. Partner Abuse. 2012;**3**:406-428

[92] Fekkes M, Pijpers FIM, Fredriks AM, Vogels T, Verloove-Vanhorick SP. Do bullied children get Ill, or do Ill children get bullied? A prospective cohort study on the relationship between bullying and health-related symptoms. Pediatrics. 2006;**117**(5):1568-1574

[93] Walsh SD, Molcho M, Craig W, Harel-Fisch Y, Huynh Q, Kukaswadia A, et al. Physical and emotional health problems experienced by youth engaged in physical fighting and weapon carrying. PLoS One. 2013;**8**(2):e56403

[94] Hertz MF, Everett Jones S, Barrios L, David-Ferdon C, Holt M. Association between bullying victimization and health risk behaviors among high school students in the United States. The Journal of School Health. 2015;**85**(12):833-842

[95] Beran T, Stanton L, Hetherington R, Mishna F, Shariff S. Development of the bullying and health experiences scale. Interactive Journal of Medical Research. 2012;**1**(2):e13

[96] Kshirsagar VY, Agarwal R, Bavdekar SB. Bullying in schools: Prevalence and short-term impact. Indian Pediatrics. 2007;**44**(1):25-28

[97] Barzilay S, Brunstein Klomek A, Apter A, Carli V, Wasserman C, Hadlaczky G, et al. Bullying victimization and suicide ideation and behavior among adolescents in Europe: A 10-country study. The Journal of Adolescent Health. 2017;**61**(2):179-186

[98] Holt MK, Kaufman Kantor G, Finkelhor D. Parent/child concordance about bullying involvement and family characteristics related to bullying and peer victimization. Journal of School Violence. 2008;**8**(1):42-63

[99] Renouf AG, Harter S. Low self-worth and anger as components of the depressive experience in young adolescents. Development and Psychopathology. 1990;**2**(3):293-310

[100] Rutter M. Achievements and challenges in the biology of environmental effects. Proceedings of the National Academy of Sciences of the United States of America. 2012;**109**(Suppl. 2):17149-17153

[101] Meaney MJ. Maternal care, gene expression, and the transmission of individual differences in stress reactivity across generations. Annual Review of Neuroscience. 2001;**24**:1161-1192

[102] Liu D, Diorio J, Tannenbaum B, Caldji C, Francis D, Freedman A, et al. Maternalcare, hippocampalglucocorticoid receptors, and hypothalamic-pituitary-adrenal responses to stress. Science. 1997;**277**(5332):1659-1662

[103] Lacey RE, Kumari M, McMunn A. Parental separation in childhood and adult inflammation: The importance of material and psychosocial pathways. Psychoneuroendocrinology. 2013;**38**(11):2476-2484

[104] Coelho R, Viola T, Walss-Bass C, Brietzke E, Grassi-Oliveira R. Childhood maltreatment and inflammatory markers: A systematic review. Acta Psychiatrica Scandinavica. 2014;**129**(3):180-192

[105] Miller AH, Maletic V, Raison CL. Inflammation and its discontents: The role of cytokines in the pathophysiology of major depression. Biological Psychiatry. 2009;**65**(9):732-741

[106] Soares S, Rocha V, Kelly-Irving M, Stringhini S, Fraga S. Adverse childhood events and health biomarkers: A systematic review. Frontiers Public Health. 2021;**9**:649-825

[107] Copeland WE, Wolke D, Lereya ST, Shanahan L, Worthman C, Costello EJ. Childhood bullying involvement predicts low-grade systemic inflammation into adulthood. Proceedings of the National Academy of Sciences of the United States of America. 2014;**111**(21):7570-7575

[108] Shalev I, Moffitt TE, Sugden K, Williams B, Houts RM, Danese A, et al. Exposure to violence during childhood is associated with telomere erosion from 5 to 10 years of age: A longitudinal study. Molecular Psychiatry. 2013;**18**(5):576-581

[109] Östberg V, Låftman SB, Modin B, Lindfors P. Bullying as a

stressor in mid-adolescent girls and boys-associations with perceived stress, recurrent pain, and salivary cortisol. International Journal of Environmental Research and Public Health. 2018;**15**(2):364

[110] Hajat A, Nurius P, Song C. Differing trajectories of adversity over the life course: Implications for adult health and well-being. Child Abuse and Neglect. 2020;**102**:104392

[111] Mackenbach JP. Persistence of social inequalities in modern welfare states: Explanation of a paradox. Scandinavian Journal of Public Health. 2017;**45**(2):113-120

[112] Kelly-Irving M. Allostatic load: How stress in childhood affects life-course health outcomes. Health Foundation. 2019. Available from: https://www.health.org.uk/publications/allostatic-load

[113] Yule K, Houston J, Grych J. Resilience in children exposed to violence: A meta-analysis of protective factors across ecological contexts. Clinical Child and Family Psychology Review. 2019;**22**(3):406-431

[114] Fergus S, Zimmerman MA. Adolescent resilience: A framework for understanding healthy development in the face of risk. Annual Review of Public Health. 2005;**26**:399-419

[115] Fritz J, de Graaff AM, Caisley H, van Harmelen AL, Wilkinson PO. A systematic review of amenable resilience factors that moderate and/or mediate the relationship between childhood adversity and mental health in young people. Frontiers in Psychiatry. 2018;**9**:230

[116] Pettoello-Mantovani M, Pop TL, Mestrovic J, Ferrara P, Giardino I, Carrasco-Sanz A, et al. Fostering resilience in children: The essential role of healthcare professionals and families. Journal of Pediatrics. 2019;**205**:298-299

[117] Crandall A, Broadbent E, Stanfill M, Magnusson BM, Novilla MLB, Hanson CL, et al. The influence of adverse and advantageous childhood experiences during adolescence on young adult health. Child Abuse and Neglect. 2020;**108**:104644

[118] Zimmerman MA. Resiliency theory: A strengths-based approach to research and practice for adolescent health. Health Education and Behavior. 2013;**40**(4):381-383

[119] Narayan AJ, Rivera LM, Bernstein RE, Harris WW, Lieberman AF. Positive childhood experiences predict less psychopathology and stress in pregnant women with childhood adversity: A pilot study of the benevolent childhood experiences (BCEs) scale. Child Abuse and Neglect. 2018;**78**:19-30

[120] Crandall A, Miller JR, Cheung A, Novilla LK, Glade R, Novilla MLB, et al. ACEs and counter-ACEs: How positive and negative childhood experiences influence adult health. Child Abuse and Neglect. 2019;**96**:104089

[121] Houshyar S, Kaufman J. Resiliency in maltreated children. In: Goldstein SBRB, editor. Handbook of Resilience in Children. New York: Springer; 2005. pp. 181-200

[122] Clark H, Coll-Seck AM, Banerjee A, Peterson S, Dalglish SL, Ameratunga S, et al. A future for the world's children? A WHO-UNICEF-Lancet Commission. Lancet. 2020;**395**(10224):605-658

Chapter 4

The Impact of Second Step Child Protection Unit Teacher Training: Latent Moderated Structural Equation Modeling (SEM) Approach

Sunha Kim, Amanda B. Nickerson and Tia E. Kim

Abstract

Given the high prevalence and harmful consequences of child sexual abuse (CSA), we need to empower teachers to play a critical role in prevention/intervention efforts. We therefore explored the potential of CSA teacher training to improve preventive outcomes based on teachers' CSA knowledge. Analyzing the data from the implementation of a CSA prevention program using structural equation modeling (SEM) revealed a significant effect of CSA teacher training on improving teachers' CSA knowledge, particularly in teachers with lower prior knowledge.

Keywords: child sexual abuse, prevention, intervention, teachers, SEM

1. Introduction

Child sexual abuse (CSA) has traumatized millions of boys and girls worldwide [1]. In the United States alone, more than 57,000 child victims were reported during 2015 and it has been suggested that as many as 28% of youths aged from 14 to 17 are exposed to CSA [2–4]. The actual CSA occurrence rate may be even higher, given that only around one-third of child abuse cases are reported to authorities and CSA is considered to be greatly underreported [3, 5, 6].

These shocking statistics should be driving urgent action by administrators and policy-makers given the highly detrimental short- and long-term consequences of CSA, which include re-victimization, substance abuse, poor mental and physical health, lower academic achievement, higher school dropout levels, and suicidal ideation/attempts [3, 7–12].

As part of our effort to prevent/intervene the occurrence of CSA and address both its high prevalence rate and serious adverse consequences, we explored the possible contribution of the teachers and other school staff members who play a critical role in educating children about sexual abuse and self-protection, and who are in an excellent position to notice sudden changes in children's behavior that may indicate abuse [13, 14]. Despite their critical role and their mandatory requirement to report suspected abuse, research has shown that most teachers lack sufficient knowledge to identify potential cases of CSA and are unfamiliar with their schools' procedures for reporting their suspicions [15–17]. Furthermore, one-third of teachers underreport child abuse [18, 19].

To address any issues that teachers might have in spite of their important roles, we investigated the effect of relevant teacher training based on the findings reported in several prior studies. Previous studies of the impact of providing CSA prevention programs for teachers have shown that they result in significant increases in knowledge, opinions, and anticipated behaviors when dealing with children who have been or are being sexually abused [15, 20]. Teachers were found to have high satisfaction levels related to this specialized training, increasing both their awareness of the problem and their readiness/inclination to develop prevention/intervention plans in the future [21].

In view of the potential role of teacher training in making teachers better prepared to execute CSA prevention/intervention plans, in this study we sought to investigate whether/how teacher training can increase important teacher outcomes, represented here by teachers' CSA knowledge [22–24]. At the same time, we looked at the moderating role of teachers' preexisting knowledge, by examining the effect of teacher training on those teachers who had lower initial levels of knowledge.

For this empirical investigation, we analyzed the data from teachers who participated in the *Second Step* Children Protection Unit (CPU). CPU is a comprehensive CSA prevention program developed by the Committee for Children (CfC) (http://www.cfchildren.org/child-protection) to offer specialized teacher training on this difficult subject. We applied a series of structural equation modeling (SEM) analyses to investigate the effect of this widely accepted teacher training intervention as well as any interaction effect between the baseline (teachers' preexisting knowledge) and the intervention [25, 26]. We also investigated the association between teachers' acceptance of the CSA interventions and their CSA knowledge after the CPU teacher training.

The following research questions guided our study.

1. Does the CPU teacher training result in any improvement in teacher knowledge of CSA?

2. Does the CPU teacher training interact with teachers' prior knowledge to improve their CSA knowledge?

2. Methods

2.1 Sample and intervention

The participants consisted of 161 teachers from a randomized control study designed to evaluate CPU. These participating teachers taught students in grades PreK-5 in elementary schools in New York State and their teaching experience ranged from 1 year to more than 30 years. Participating teachers were assigned to either the intervention group or the control group. The teachers in the intervention group received the treatment by taking the CPU online teacher training, which consisted of two modules: *Policies and Procedures* (75–90 min) and *Recognize, Respond, and Report*

Abuse (45–75 min). The intervention teachers also implemented the CPU 6-week lessons with children in their classrooms. Teachers in the intervention group completed pretest/posttest measure assessing their knowledge of CSA prior to receiving the training and afterwards. The same pretest/posttest measure was administered to the teachers in the control group who did not receive the training.

2.2 Measures

Participating teachers were asked to complete the measures described below. Teachers in both the intervention and control groups completed the measure on teachers' preventive outcome in terms of knowledge.

Educators and Child Abuse Questionnaire (*ECAQ*;23): The *ECAQ* was used to assess knowledge of both CSA and policy components (e.g., reporting procedures). Out of the total of four subscales of *ECAQ*, this study examined one subscale of awareness of signs and symptoms of child abuse featuring good psychometric quality in our study settings. It has been used in several studies [16, 23, 27] to assess educators' knowledge and competence with regard to CSA and policies. The measure includes 12 items on a 5-point Likert scale ranging from *strongly agree (1) to strongly disagree (5)* (Some items are reverse-coded so that higher scores represent more knowledge) (**Table 1**).

2.3 Analysis

We analyzed the data by building a series of SEM models utilizing Mplus 8.1 [28]. Particularly, we took a latent variable moderated SEM approach to test how teachers' baseline knowledge measured at the pretest moderated the effect of the teacher training intervention on teacher knowledge at the posttest, in addition to the effect of the teacher training intervention on teacher knowledge at the posttest [29–32].

Figure 1 shows a conceptual diagram of our SEM model (Intervention Model) with our teacher training intervention (*train*: coded 0 for the control group; 1 for the intervention group), as well as the indicator variables (*awar1_1*, *awar1_2*, and *awar1_3*) for the latent teacher knowledge at the pretest (*awar1*) and those (*awar2_1*, *awar2_2*, and *awar2_3*) for the latent teacher knowledge at the posttest (*awar2*). The latent moderation (aka, interaction) model included the interaction term (*awar1tr*) by adopting the latent moderator variable (*awar1*) and the teacher training intervention (*train*).

In addition, we calculated simple slopes in order to investigate further the latent moderation effect with focused attention on the intervention effect on teachers with lower initial knowledge. Specifically, the simple slopes were assessed at three values of the moderator (teacher knowledge construct at pretest: *awar1*) below, at, and above the baseline average (*MODLO*, *MOD0*, and *MODHI*, respectively). Moreover, we explored the latent interaction effect across the value range of the latent moderator (*awar1*) beyond its three specific values by producing a series of LOOP plots.

	ECAQ (Pretest)	ECAQ (Posttest)
Reliability (α)	0.77	0.86

Table 1.
Reliability of measures.

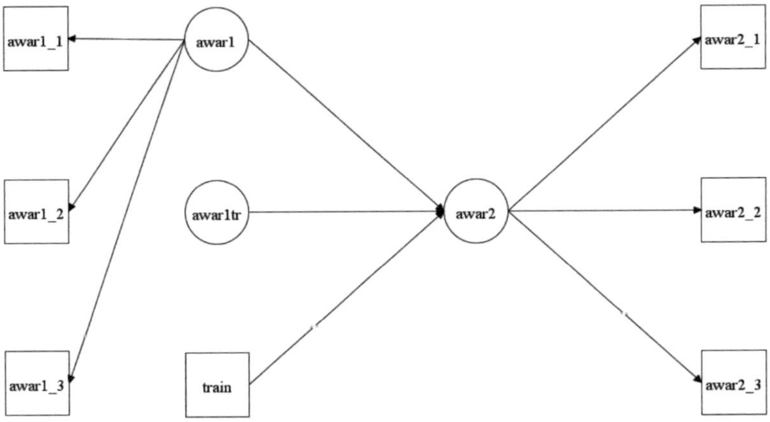

Figure 1.
Conceptual diagram of SEM model.

3. Results

As the results presented in **Table 2** indicate, our Intervention Model had acceptable fit statistics: $X^2(10) = 15.48, p > 0.05$; RMSEA = 0.06 (<0.08); CFI = 0.99 (>0.95); and TLI = 0.97 (>0.95) [31, 33–36].

Figure 2 presents the conceptual model for the Intervention Model with parameter estimates from the *Mplus* outputs. The CPU teacher training (*train*) was effective in improving teacher knowledge (*awar2*) ($\beta = 0.51, p < 0.01$). There was a significant positive effect of teacher prior knowledge (*awar1*) on teacher knowledge at the posttest (*awar2*) ($\beta = 0.54, p < 0.05$).

On the other hand, we detected insignificant interaction/moderation effect (*awar1tr*) with $\beta = -0.20, p = 0.40$. To understand more detailed implications of the moderation/interaction effect, we reviewed simple slope results, which were estimated in the sections of the New/Additional Parameters in **Table 3**. We identified significant effects of the teacher training on improving teachers' CSA knowledge at three specific values: below, at, and above the mean ($\beta = 0.59, p = 0.00$, $\beta = 0.51, p = 0.00$, $\beta = 0.44, p = 0.00$, respectively). Among these three estimates for simple slopes, we found a greater magnitude at the lower moderator value (*MODLO*) compared with two other values (*MOD0* and *MODHI*).

To visually represent how the teacher training effect was moderated by teacher knowledge at the pretest, we produced LOOP Plots. **Figure 3** shows the range of the moderator values (*awar1*) along the x-axis for which the effect of teacher training

Fit indices	
Chi-square (*df*)	15.48 (*10*), $p = 0.12$
RMSEA	0.06
CFI	0.99
TLI	0.97

RMSEA, root mean square error of approximation; CFI, comparative fit index; TLI, Tucker-Lewis index.

Table 2.
Fit statistics.

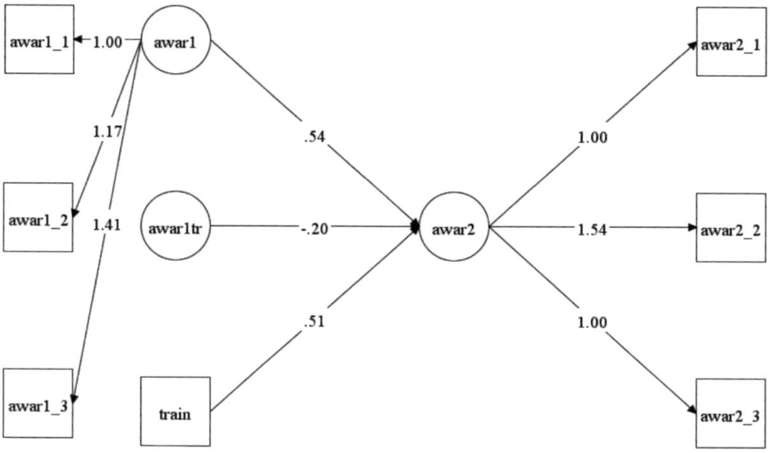

Figure 2.
Parameter estimates for SEM model.

	Estimate	S.E.	*p*
AWAR1 BY			
AWAR1_1	1.00	0.00	999.00
AWAR1_2	1.17	0.18	0.00
AWAR1_3	1.41	0.33	0.00
AWAR 2 BY			
AWAR2_1	1.00	0.00	999.00
AWAR2_2	1.54	0.27	0.00
AWAR2_3	1.00	0.11	0.00
AWAR 2 ON			
AWAR1	0.54	0.27	0.04
AWAR1TR	−0.20	0.24	0.40
TRAIN	0.51	0.09	0.00
New/additional parameters			
MODLO	0.59	0.14	0.00
MOD0	0.51	0.09	0.00
MODHI	0.44	0.11	0.00

Table 3.
Parameter estimates for SEM model.

(*train*) is significant. The straight line shown in red represents the estimated moderator function and the blue curves represent the confidence intervals. As the graph shows, the intervention effect has a greater positive value with decreasing values of baseline teacher knowledge. This suggests that the effect of the teacher training tended to be more pronounced among teachers with lower baseline scores, as would be expected.

In **Figure 4**, the bold blue line (TX1) displays the estimate for preventive knowledge average at the posttest among the intervention group teachers, with the bold

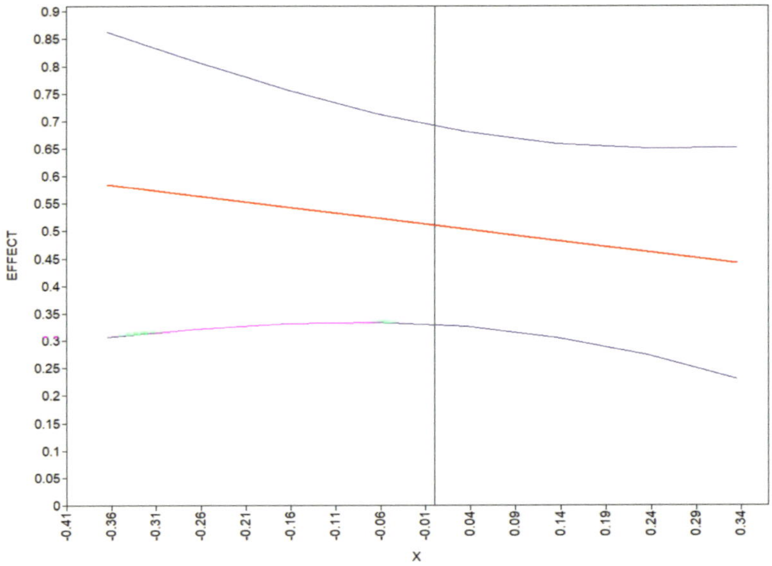

Figure 3.
Estimated moderator function and confidence interval.

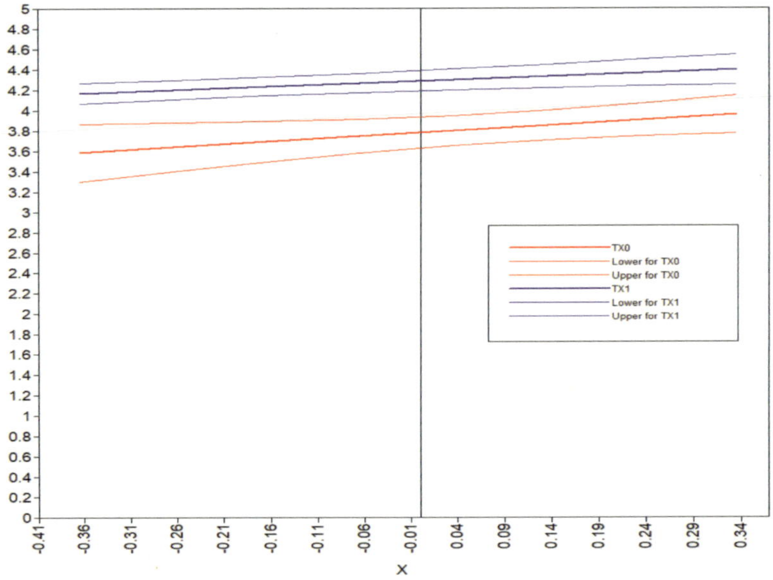

Figure 4.
The posttest (teacher knowledge) means as a function of baseline for the intervention and the control groups.

red line (TX0) representing that among the control group teachers. The effect of the teacher training denotes the gap between TX1 and TX0. The gap widens at the lower baseline scores, while narrowing at the higher baseline scores. Corresponding to those estimates for the above mentioned simple slopes, LOOP Plot results revealed that the CPU teacher training was more effective among teachers with lower CSA awareness at pretest.

4. Significance

Given the prevalence and serious adverse outcomes of CSA persistently observed despite international efforts such as the declaration of the Rights of the Child by the United Nations [37], we sought to evaluate the effectiveness of efforts to prevent and intervene to ameliorate the effects of CSA by focusing on teachers as they not only have great accessibility to children but also expertise in child education/development [13, 20]. To help teachers, who unfortunately have felt unprepared and unsure of how to intervene/protect their students from those who might be abusing them [17, 38], we explored the potential role of teacher training for improving teachers' preventive outcomes of knowledge.

By analyzing empirical data from an implementation of the CPU, we found a significant effect of CPU teacher training on improving teachers' preventive knowledge. These results are in accordance with those reported in prior studies of the positive association between teacher training and teacher outcomes such as CSA knowledge, attitudes, and confidence [15, 21]. Crucially, we found the effect of CPU teacher training was more pronounced for teachers with the lower baseline scores in terms of teacher knowledge. Our findings based on empirical data for elementary school teachers from the years 2017–2018 contribute to the field of CSA prevention programs by addressing concerns that existing evaluation studies of CSA prevention programs in this fast-moving field have become outdated [39–41].

Given these findings, we urge administrators and policy-makers to devote more funding to efforts to develop and/or offer more teacher training opportunities, including investing in CPU teacher training. Our results show that these teacher training programs would possibly help teachers confront this uncomfortable issue and deal with the consequences, particularly those who started with relatively low levels of CSA knowledge. This is important as it may empower teachers to respond and intervene more effectively.

To respond to the concerns teachers expressed regarding their lack of knowledge and competency, despite their critical role for CSA prevention/intervention efforts [15, 17], we sought to strengthen teachers' individual preventive outcomes via teacher training. Also, our other studies showed the potential effects of teacher training on other preventive outcomes for teachers as well as students' preventive outcomes [42, 43]. However, one limitation of our approach is that we only included educators working in schools. Given CSA occurrence in various organizations, such as sporting institutes and religious organizations, importantly, professionals, who are responsible for child-care and build rapport with the children across varying institutions, need to be equipped with an awareness of CSA signals and symptoms and knowledge to report suspected CSA cases [44–46]. Future studies should extend the findings of this study to develop and/or improve training that will empower child-care professionals across all such organizations with preventative knowledge to protect children from the threat of CSA. Providing networking opportunities via the training sessions for these child-care professionals could also contribute by building a community of child-care professionals where these professionals work together to develop more comprehensive prevention solutions.

Acknowledgements

This work was supported by the Committee for Children, Seattle, WA.

Conflict of interest

The authors declare no conflict of interest. Dr. Tia Kim is employed by the Committee for Children.

Author details

Sunha Kim[1*], Amanda B. Nickerson[1] and Tia E. Kim[2]

1 CSEP, GSE, University at Buffalo, Buffalo, NY, USA

2 Committee for Children, Seattle, WA, USA

*Address all correspondence to: sunhakim@buffalo.edu

References

[1] Barth J, Bermetz L, Heim E, Trelle S, Tonia T. The current prevalence of child sexual abuse worldwide: A systematic review and meta-analysis. International Journal of Public Health. 2013;**58**(3):469-483

[2] Crea TM, Easton SD, Florio J, Barth RP. Externalizing behaviors among adopted children: A longitudinal comparison of preadoptive childhood sexual abuse and other forms of maltreatment. Child Abuse & Neglect. 2018;**82**:192-200

[3] Finkelhor D, Turner H, Hamby SL, Ormrod R. Polyvictimization: Children's Exposure to Multiple Types of Violence, Crime, and Abuse. National Survey of Children's Exposure to Violence. Washington, DC: US Government Printing Office; 2011

[4] U.S. Department of Health & Human Services, Administration for Children and Families, Administration on Children, Youth and Families, Children's Bureau. Child Maltreatment 2015. 2015. Available from: https://www.acf.hhs.gov/sites/default/files/cb/cm2015.pdf

[5] Kellogg N. The evaluation of sexual abuse in children. Pediatrics. 2005;**116**(2):506-512

[6] Sedlak AJ, Mettenburg J, Basena M, Petta I, McPherson K, Greene A, et al. Fourth National Incidence Study of Child Abuse and Neglect (NIS-4): Report to Congress. Washington, DC: U.S. Department of Health and Human Services, Administration for Children and Families; 2010

[7] Badmaeva VD. Consequences of sexual abuse in children and adolescents. Neuroscience and Behavioral Physiology. 2011;**41**(3):259-262. DOI: 10.1007/s11055-011-9409-6

[8] Boden JM, Horwood LJ, Fergusson DM. Exposure to childhood sexual and physical abuse and subsequent educational achievement outcomes. Child Abuse & Neglect. 2007;**31**(10):1101-1114

[9] Frothingham TE, Hobbs CJ, Wynne JM, Yee L, Goyal A, Wadsworth DJ. Follow up study eight years after diagnosis of sexual abuse. Archives of Disease in Childhood. 2000;**83**(2):132-134

[10] Lown EA, Nayak MB, Korcha RA, Greenfield TK. Child physical and sexual abuse: A comprehensive look at alcohol consumption patterns, consequences, and dependence from the National Alcohol Survey. Alcoholism: Clinical and Experimental Research. 2011;**35**(2):317-325. DOI: 10.1111/j.1530-0277.2010.01347.x

[11] Messman-Moore TL, Long PJ. The role of childhood sexual abuse sequelae in the sexual revictimization of women: An empirical review and theoretical reformulation. Clinical Psychology Review. 2003;**23**(4):537-571. DOI: 10.1016/S0272-7358(02)00203-9

[12] Morrow AS, Villodas MT. Direct and indirect pathways from adverse childhood experiences to high school dropout among high-risk adolescents. Journal of Research on Adolescence. 2018;**28**(2):327-341

[13] Nickerson AB, Heath MA, Graves LA. School-based interventions for children impacted by sexual abuse. In: Paludi M, DenMark FL, editors. Victims of Sexual Assault and Abuse: Resources and Responses for Individuals and Families, Vol. 2: Cultural, Community, Educational

and Advocacy Responses. Santa Barbara, CA: Praeger; 2010. pp. 77-99

[14] Renk K, Liljequist L, Steinberg A, Bosco G, Phares V. Prevention of child sexual abuse: Are we doing enough? Trauma, Violence, & Abuse. 2002;**3**(1): 68-84

[15] Kleemeir C, Webb C, Hazzard A, Pohl J. Child sexual abuse prevention: Evaluation of a teacher training model. Child Abuse & Neglect. 1988;**12**:555-561

[16] Kenny MC. Teachers' attitudes toward and knowledge of child maltreatment. Child Abuse & Neglect. 2004;**28**:1311-1319

[17] Marquez-Flores MM, Marquez-Hernandez VV, Granados-Gamez G. Teacher's knowledge and beliefs about child sexual abuse. Journal of Child Sexual Abuse: Research Treatment and Program Innovations for Victims, Survivors, & Offenders. 2016;**25**:538-555

[18] Walsh K, Bridgstock R, Farrell A, Rassafiani M, Schweitzer R. Case, teacher and school characteristics influencing teachers' detection and reporting of child physical abuse and neglect: Results from an Australian survey. Child Abuse & Neglect. 2008;**32**:983-993

[19] Webster SW, O'Toole RO, O'Toole AW, Lucal B. Overreporting and underreporting of child abuse: Teachers' use of professional discretion. Child Abuse & Neglect. 2005;**29**:1281-1296. DOI: 10.1016/j.chiabu.2004.02.007

[20] Rheingold AA, Zajac K, Chapman JE, Patton M, de Arellano M, Saunders B, et al. Child sexual abuse prevention training for childcare professionals: An independent multi-site randomized controlled trial of stewards of children. Prevention Science. 2015;**16**(3):374-385

[21] Gushwa M, Bernier J, Robinson D. Advancing child sexual abuse prevention in schools: An exploration of the effectiveness of the Enough! online training program for K-12 teachers. Journal of Child Sexual Abuse. 2019;**28**(2):144-159. DOI: 10.1080/10538712.2018.1477000

[22] Bear GG, Yang C, Pell M, Gaskins C. Validation of a brief measure of teachers' perceptions of school climate: Relations to student achievement and suspensions. Learning Environment Research. 2014;**17**:339-354. DOI: 10.1007/s10984-014-9162-1

[23] Kenny M. Child abuse reporting: Teachers' perceived deterrents. Child Abuse & Neglect. 2001;**25**(1):81-92

[24] Walsh K, Rassafiani M, Matthews B, Farrell A, Butler D. Teachers' attitudes toward reporting child sexual abuse: Problems with existing research leading to new scale development. Journal of Child Sexual Abuse. 2010;**19**:310-336. DOI: 10.1080/10538711003781392

[25] Brown C, Wang W, Kellam S, Petras H, Toyinbo P, Poduska J, et al. Methods for testing theory and evaluating impact in randomized field trials: Intent-to-treat analyses for integrating the perspectives of person, place, and time. Drug and Alcohol Dependence. 2008;**95**(Supplement 1):S74-S104

[26] Kellam S, Brown C, Poduska J, Ialongo N, Petras H, Wang W, et al. Effects of a universal classroom behavior management program in first and second grades on young adult behavioral, psychiatric, and social outcomes. Drug and Alcohol Dependence. 2008;**95**(Supplement 1):S5-S28

[27] Kenny M, McEachern A. Reporting of suspected child abuse: A pilot comparison of middle and high school

counselors and principals. Journal of Child Sexual Abuse. 2002;**11**(2):59-75

[28] Muthén LK, Muthén BO. Mplus User's Guide. 8th ed. Los Angeles, CA: Muthén & Muthén; 1998-2017

[29] Kline RB. Principles and Practice of Structural Equation Modeling. 3rd ed. New York: Guilford; 2011

[30] Muthén BO, Muthén LK, Asparouhov T. Regression and Mediation Analysis Using Mplus. Los Angeles, CA: Muthén & Muthén; 2017

[31] Schumacker RE, Lomax RG. A Beginners' Guide to Structural Equation Modeling. 4th ed. New York: Routledge; 2010

[32] Maslowsky J, Jager J, Hemken D. Estimating and interpreting latent variable interactions: A tutorial for applying the latent moderated structural equations method. International Journal of Behavioral Development. 2015;**39**(1):87-96

[33] Browne MW, Cudeck R. Alternative ways of assessing model fit. In: Bollen KA, Long JS, editors. Testing Structural Equation Models. Beverly Hills, CA: Sage; 1993. pp. 136-162

[34] Hooper D, Coughlan J, Mullen MR. Structural equation modeling: Guidelines for determining model fit. Electronic Journal of Business Research Methods. 2008;**6**:53-60

[35] Raykov T, Marcoulidies GA. A First Course in Structural Equation Modeling. Mahwah, NJ: Erlbaum; 2000

[36] Yu CY, Muthén BO. Evaluation of Model Fit Indices for Latent Variable Models with Categorical and Continuous Outcomes (Technical Report). Los Angeles, CA: University of California at Los Angeles, Graduate School of Education and Information Studies; 2001

[37] United Nations. Convention on the rights of the child. 1989. Retrieved from: https://www.ohchr.org/en/professionalinterest/pages/crc.aspx

[38] Hinkelman L, Bruno M. Identification and reporting of child sexual abuse: The role of elementary school professionals. The Elementary School Journal. 2008;**108**(5):376-391

[39] Babatsikos G. Parents' knowledge, attitudes and practices about preventing child sexual abuse: A literature review. Child Abuse Review: Journal of the British Association for the Study and Prevention of Child Abuse and Neglect. 2010;**19**(2):107-129

[40] Tutty LM. Listen to the children: Kids' impressions of who do you tell™. Journal of Child Sexual Abuse. 2014;**23**:17-37. DOI: 10.1080/10538712.2013.841790

[41] Walsh K, Zwi K, Woolfenden S, Shlonsky A. School-based Education Programmes for the Prevention of Child Sexual Abuse. Hoboken, NJ: John Wiley & Sons; 2015. DOI: 10.1002/14651858.CD00430.pub3

[42] Manges ME, Nickerson AB. Student knowledge gain following the Second Step Child Protection Unit: The influence of treatment integrity. Prevention Science. 2020;**21**(8):1037-1047

[43] Nickerson A, Kim S, Dudley M, Livingston JA, Manges M. Longitudinal impact of the Second Step Child Protection Unit on teacher knowledge, attitude, and climate. Children and Youth Services Review. 2021;**123**:105892

[44] Finkelhor D, Shattuck A, Turner HA, Hamby SL. The lifetime prevalence of

child sexual abuse and sexual assault assessed in late adolescence. Journal of Adolescent Health. 2014;**55**(3):329-333. DOI: 10.1016/j.jadohealth.2013.12.026

[45] Nurse AM. Coaches and child sexual abuse prevention training: Impact on knowledge, confidence, and behavior. Children and Youth Services Review. 2018;**88**:395-400

[46] Ratliff L, Watson J. A descriptive analysis of public school educators arrested for sex offenses. Journal of Child Sexual Abuse. 2014;**23**(2):217-228

Chapter 5

What Accommodations Do Courts Provide for Abused Children with Communication Disabilities? A Legal Scoping Review

Juan Bornman, Robyn White and Ensa Johnson

Abstract

Children with disabilities are at higher risk for becoming victims of violence and sexual abuse than peers without disabilities. Despite this, very few of these cases are heard in court due to a plethora of reasons. In the rare event that they do, the court appears to be unaware and unable to efficiently provide accommodations that would allow these children to testify and obtain justice. The aim of this legal scoping review was to identify the range of documented court accommodations to enable abused children with communication disabilities to testify in court. The legal scoping review methodology developed by White et al. (2021) was used to search the extant evidence related to court accommodations for children with communication disabilities across electronic social sciences databases (i.e., PubMed, CINAHL, The Cochrane Library and PscyInfo) and law databases (i.e., Hein Online, Lexis Nexis, Sabinet and Saflii). Results describe the available accommodations used across different countries and jurisdictions.

Keywords: accommodations, court, sexual abuse, children with disabilities, law, witness, victim

1. Introduction

Children—all children—should be seen, heard, respected, and cherished, not hidden, silenced, abused and neglected. The umbrella term “child abuse” includes sexual abuse, physical abuse, emotional abuse, neglect and exploitation of children [1] and affects more than one billion children globally—half of the children in the world [2]. Hence it is safe to say that child abuse is one of the most prevalent challenges affecting modern society.

Certain factors appear to increase children’s risk of abuse even further, and these can be related to either the environment, or to adults in the child’s life (including parents) or to the children themselves. Regarding the environment it has been reported that children from impoverished neighborhoods who live in poverty have a heightened risk [3] as are children with smaller social networks and those who experience greater social isolation [4].

Regarding adult factors, research on parenting has noted that social and economic instability and difficulty, parental mental illness and substance abuse are strongly correlated to child abuse [5]. Parental mental illness and substance abuse [5] as well as low parental involvement also increase the risk. Furthermore, overly strict parenting styles might be linked to an increase risk of child abuse too [6]. Parents of children with disabilities in particular have increased financial, physical and emotional responsibilities related to caring for their child's needs which may result in heightened mental and emotional stress [7] and eventually burn out and neglect [8, 9].

Apart from parents, children also face the risk of "professional perpetrators" such as teachers, priests and sports coaches (i.e., adults who use their work with children and seek out contexts to enable abuse) [10, 11]. In several East African countries for example, teachers are known for verbal and physical abuse [12, 13].

Regarding child factors it appears as if younger children who are more dependent on others, (including parents) for their daily care, experience the highest rates of child abuse [14]. Apart from age, other child factors may also heighten their risk, namely the presence of a disability: more specifically intellectual disability [15, 16], autism spectrum disorder (ASD) [17] and communication disability [18], as well as emotional and/or behavioral disabilities (i.e., anxiety and depression, Attention Deficit Hyperactivity Disorder (ADHD), aggressive behavior and rule breaking behavior) [19, 20]. A large meta-analysis estimated that children with disabilities were at three to five times higher risk of abuse than same-aged peers without disabilities [21]. Additional factors that are linked to disability and that increases the risk for abuse is the fact that these children are trained to be compliant (e.g., to facilitate the ease of caregiving due to high dependence on others for caregiving, often involving intimate activities such as toileting and bathing) [4]. Moreover, these children are typically dependent on support in their everyday lives from a range of service providers such as social workers, taxi/bus drivers, health care workers, personal assistants and other professionals, which also increases their exposure to multiple potential perpetrators [22, 23].

Additionally, it should be noted that the risk of child abuse increases exponentially with the cumulative number of risk factors experienced by a child [15]. For example, a combination of intellectual disability and ASD increases risk [17] as does intellectual disability and communication disability [24]. Barron and colleagues [25] reported that individuals with severe and complex disabilities, are at increased risk due to the potential communication barriers challenges they experience. Children with disabilities are often victims of polyvictimization as they experience several types of abuse (e.g., sexual, emotional and physical abuse) with repeated episodes when compared to their peers without disabilities [26]. This type of polyvictimization also tends to intensify if the abuse continues over time, negatively impacting on the child's well-being and quality of life [27]. Moreover, this abuse is often committed by perpetrators who are known, familiar and trusted partners [28]—not stranger abuse.

Furthermore, it should be highlighted that children typically face the added challenges of not being believed when they try to disclose abuse. This increases their risk of becoming repeat victims. For example, a third of parents in an Australian study stated that that they would not believe a child who disclosed sexual abuse [10]. It is thus hardly surprising that a recent Scandinavian study that examined police records as a possible methodology for determining abuse prevalence rates (as abuse is a criminal offense) discarded this methodology as it found a general absence of police records involving children with disabilities [29].

In addition to not being believed, children might also experience communication challenges that negatively impact on detecting or disclosing the abuse as well as on reporting it (e.g., to social workers or the police) and ultimately on testifying in court. These challenges might be related to the children's age (younger children may not yet have the needed language due to a restricted vocabulary or unintelligible speech due to the presence of articulation errors or normal phonetical processes) or due to disability (disability may result in speech that is difficult to understand, or it may limit language proficiency to clearly describe the abuse situation) [30].

Addressing childhood abuse requires a systemic approach, starting with primary intervention which entails interventions aimed at preventing abuse from happening in the first place [31] to secondary prevention which includes interventions aimed at preventing further abuse from occurring [32] and finally tertiary prevention which includes interventions aimed at decreasing the effects of abuse, such as rehabilitation and medical treatment for children [31]. Courts have a role to play in secondary prevention as perpetrators often have little or no fear for the consequences of their acts [33, 34]. Besides, perpetrators see their victims as vulnerable as they know that very few cases of childhood abuse, and even less of childhood abuse that involves children with disabilities are successfully prosecuted, and hence they exploit this vulnerability [35]. Child victims often regard courts as unapproachable, with a range of legal formalities, complex rules, and practices and formal (unfamiliar) legal language that make it difficult to navigate the court proceedings. Even formal court attire (e.g., wigs and gowns) is typically reported as being intimidating [36].

Therefore, the current study aimed to investigate which accommodations have been afforded to abused children with communication disabilities across the world to enable them to participate in court. This is seen as a way of strengthening secondary abuse prevention initiatives by bringing perpetrators to justice while also affording children with disabilities the opportunity to be accommodated to participate equally without any form of discrimination.

2. Method

The current research used data mining, and specifically the clustering technique (i.e., extrapolating new knowledge from previously collected data by grouping data together based on different demographics) [37]. The data collected in the original legal scoping review, which was the first of its kind to use that specific legal scoping review methodology at the time of publication [38], focused on court accommodations for both adults and children with severe communication disabilities and included both the accused and victims. For the purpose of this research, the original data was clustered to only focus on children, and to only focus on child victims (described as "witness" as the victim will participate in the justice system as a witness [39], thereby tightening the focus of the broader original search significantly).

In order to answer the research question, *What accommodations have been afforded to abused children with communication disabilities across the world to enable them to participate equally in court without any form of discrimination?* a legal scoping review was conducted [38]. This methodology acknowledges the nexus of social sciences and law, and hence combined the scoping review framework [40, 41] commonly used in social sciences with the steps suggested for a systematic review of legal doctrine [42]. As such, a legal scoping review can document existing evidence of a specific legal topic by describing what has been written about the topic, and how it has been examined to date, while also providing the necessary evidence to support a central claim, for example, the type and range of court accommodations that should be provided to children with disabilities. Moreover, it could assist courts by lending credibility to the process and reducing any perception of bias about their decisions [38]. The five steps proposed in the legal scoping review methodology are: i) identify and state the research question; ii) identify and define the studies related to legal cases, laws, and treaties; iii) select relevant studies; iv) chart and weigh the data (e.g., in terms of regency, citation frequency, precedential status) and v) conduct the analysis and report the results.

2.1 Identify and state the research question

The legal scoping review methodology commences with a clearly articulated research question, preferably using the PIO (Population, Intervention, Outcome) framework [43], as this guides the scope of the research and facilitates the identification of relevant information as shown in **Table 1**. Therefore, the main research question, *What accommodations* (Intervention) *have been afforded to abused children with communication disabilities across the world* (Population) *to enable them to participate equally in court without any form of discrimination* (Outcome), was supplemented by two specific sub-questions related to this population, irrespective of the country in which they reside:

1. Which sources typically document court accommodations for abused children with disabilities?

2. What is the nature of these accommodations? (In what countries are they provided? Do they cite international or national law? How many specific cases do they mention? What types of court proceedings, (e.g., criminal, civil, family), are most frequently mentioned?)

2.2 Identify and define the studies and legal cases

Clear and replicable processes were set at the start to increase data reliability [38]. The databases that were identified and selected in the social sciences were PubMed, CINAHL, the Cochrane Library and PsycInfo, while Hein Online, Lexis Nexis, Sabinet and Saflii were selected in the legal field. Thereafter, a comprehensive and systematic literature search was done using keywords based on the PIO framework (**Table 2**) with truncation (*) and Boolean operators AND and OR to link the population to the intervention and outcomes in the search.

2.3 Select relevant studies

For the current study, we clustered the information originally used for the Population (by reanalyzing it to only focus on children and child victims) while the rest remained the same, namely all publications that were available in English, that had been published between 2006 (which marks the adoption of the CRPD) and December 2019, and that focused on court accommodations for abused children with disabilities. As we reviewed the abstracts, we engaged in an iterative process of refining our inclusion and exclusion criteria (see **Table 2**), based on the PIO framework mentioned earlier.

Figure 1 outlines of the study selection process in accordance with the Preferred Reporting Items for Systematic Review and Meta-Analyses (PRISMA) statement [46].

Descriptive information about articles					Population	Outcomes		
#	Authors	Year	Source	Country	Children's type of disability	International /national law	Type of court	Specific law(s) mentioned
1	Backstrom, J.C.	2016	Law journal article	• USA	• Not specified	National	Not specified	• Minnesota State Legislature, 2015
2	Benedet, J. Grant, I.	2012	Law journal article	• Canada, • South Africa • England	• Intellectual • Physical • Multiple	National	Criminal	• Section 486.1 of the Code, Section 486.2(1) of the Code • Section 16 of Youth Justice and Evidence Act, 1999 • Section 170A (1) of the Criminal Law (Sexual Of- fences and Related Matters) Act
3	BenZeev, N., Lerner, N., Klein, Y.	2014	Book chapter	• Israel	• Intellectual • Physical • Communication	National and International	Criminal	• Investigation and Testimony Procedures (Adaptation to Persons with Mental or Psychological Disability) Law, 2005
4	Bornman, J.	2014	Book chapter	• South Africa	• Communication	National and International	Not specified	• CRC • African Charter on the Rights and Welfare of the Child • CRPD • Constitution of the Republic of South Africa (including the Bill of Rights) • Children's Act 38, 2005 • Criminal Law (Sexual Offenses and Related Matters) Amendment Act, 2007 • Mental Health Care Act 17, 2002
5	Bryen, D.N. Wickman, C.	2014	Book chapter	• USA	• Communication • Physical • ASD	National	Criminal, State, Supreme, Court of Appeal	• California rule of evidence 701, • Section 387 of the Judiciary Law of the state of New York
6	Carter, E., Boezaart, T.	2016	Law journal article	• South Africa	• Not specified	National and International	Children's, Criminal Civil	• United Nation's Declaration on the Rights of Mentally Retarded Persons, 1971 • Declaration on the Rights of Disabled Persons, 1975

	Descriptive information about articles				Population	Outcomes		
#	Authors	Year	Source	Country	Children's type of disability	International /national law	Type of court	Specific law(s) mentioned
								• CRC • CRPD • Children's Act 38, 2005
7	Cooper, P.,Dando, C.,Ormerod, T., Mattison, M., Marchant, R., Milne, R., Bull, R.	2018	Law journal article	• UK	• Not specified	National and International	Not specified	• Youth Justice and Criminal Evidence Act, 1999 • Mental Health Act, 1983
8	Cusack, A.	2017	Law journal article	• Ireland	• Intellectual	National	Criminal	• Criminal Evidence Act • Criminal Law (Sexual Offenses) Act, 2017
9	Doak, J., Doak, L.	2017	Law journal article	• Ireland • England • Wales	• Intellectual • Physical • Communication	National	Criminal	• Criminal Justice Act 2003 as an exception to the hearsay rule • Youth Justice and Criminal Evidence Act (YJCEA), 1999
10	Edwards, C., Harold, G., Kilcommins, S.	2012	Research paper	• Ireland	• Intellectual	National and International	Criminal	• Section 29(1) of the Criminal Evidence Act, 1992 • Criminal Justice Act, 2006 • Criminal Procedure Act, 2010 • YJCEA 1999 • Disability Act, 2005 in Ireland • Disability Discrimination Act (DDA), 2005 in the UK • Americans with Disabilities Act (ADA), 1990 • New South Wales Evidence Act, 1995 • CRPD—Article 13
11	Flynn, E.	2016	Book chapter	• South Africa • USA • UK • Ireland • Bulgaria	• Intellectual • Physical • Communication • Hearing	National and International	Criminal SA Equality Court European Court of Human	• The Promotion of Equality and Prevention of Unfair Discrimination Act of 2000 South Africa • American Disabilities Act (ADA), 1990 • Article 6 of the European Convention

Descriptive information about articles					Population	Outcomes		
#	Authors	Year	Source	Country	Children's type of disability	International /national law	Type of court	Specific law(s) mentioned
							Rights High	• Mental Capacity Act, 2005 in England and Wales • Section 60 of the Assisted Decision-Making (Capacity) Bill
12	Hepner, I., Woodward, M., Stewart, J.	2015	Multi-disciplinary journal article	• Australia	• Not specified	National and International	Criminal	• CRPD—Article 13 • YJCEA, 1999 in the UK • Australian Law Reform Commission, 2009
13	Larcher, J.	2014	Book chapter	• UK	• Not specified	National	Not specified	• YJCEA, 1999 • Coroners and Justice Act, 2009
14	Malunga, B., Kanyongolo, N. Mweso, N.	2017	Law journal article	• Malawi	• Not specified	National and International	Criminal	• CRPD—Article 13 • Section 41 of the Malawian Constitution Section • Malawi Disability Act, 2012
15	Murphy, W.	2014	Law journal article	• USA	• Physical	National	Criminal	• Americans with Disabilities Act (ADA), 1990
16	O'Leary, C.	2016	Master's thesis	• Ireland • Australia • Israel • UK	• Not specified	National	Criminal	• CRPD—Article 13 • Criminal Evidence Act, 1992 • Criminal Law (Sexual Offenses) Act, 1993 • Evidence Act • Investigation and Testimony Procedures (Adaptation to Persons with Mental or Psychological Disability) Law, 2005 • YJCEA, 1999
17	O'Leary, C., Feely, M.	2018	Multi-disciplinary journal article	• Ireland • Australia • Israel • UK	• Not specified	National and International	Criminal	• CRPD—Article 13 • Criminal Evidence Act, 1992 • Criminal Law (Sexual Offenses) Act, 1993 • Assisted Decision Making (Capacity) Act, 2015

	Descriptive information about articles				Population	Outcomes		
#	**Authors**	**Year**	**Source**	**Country**	**Children's type of disability**	**International /national law**	**Type of court**	**Specific law(s) mentioned**
								• Evidence Act, 1995 • Investigation and Testimony Procedures (Adaptation to Persons with Mental or Psychological Disability) Law, 2005 • YJCEA, 1999
18	Pillay, A.	2012	Social science journal article	• South Africa	• Not specified	National	Criminal	• Criminal Law Amendment Act No. 10, 1997 • Criminal Law (Sexual Offenses and Related Matters) Amendment Act No. 3, 2007
19	White, R., Msipa, D.	2018	Law journal article	• South Africa	• Not specified	National	Criminal	• Criminal Procedure Act 51, 1977 • Children's Act 38, 2005 • Child Justice Act 75, 2008 • CRPD—Article 13 • Israel Act, 2005

Note: USA = United Sates of America; UK = United Kingdom (England, Wales, Scotland and Northern Ireland).

Table 1.
Descriptive characteristics of publications (N = 19).

PIO	Inclusion criteria	Exclusion criteria
P	Population: Abused children with communication disabilities who have either been victims or witnesses. Child is defined as an individual below the chronological age of eighteen years [44].	
	Children: with complex communication needs with little or no functional speech with intellectual or cognitive disabilities (can have mental illness—dual diagnosis) who had been victims of crime who had been witnesses in court who are deaf who are deaf-blind with sensory impairments with autism spectrum disorder (ASD)	Medical conditions (e.g., cardiovascular diseases, AIDS/HIV) Mental health illness that is treated with medication and defined as "... health conditions involving changes in emotion, thinking or behavior (or a combination of these). Mental illnesses are associated with distress and/or problems functioning in social, work or family activities (e.g., major depressive disorder, schizophrenia and bipolar disorder). Mental illness is treatable. The vast majority of individuals with mental illness continue to function in their daily lives." [45]. The focus of the current study is on abused children who have communication disabilities, and hence publications that reported on mental illness, mental disability and intellectual disability in the same publication were included.
I	Intervention: Court accommodations relevant to communication disability	
	Strategies, communication boards, intermediaries, court preparation officers, training, communication accommodations. Physical accommodations, wheelchair access, child-friendly rooms, separate testifying rooms.	Publications that only described barriers without referring to accommodations, were excluded. Interventions and strategies that did not focus on court accommodations for children with disabilities (e.g., attitudinal training of court officers, strategies and accommodations used at the police station).
O	Outcome: Access to justice and participation in court (in terms of types of courts and types of law)	
	Participation in court proceedings Access to justice	Accommodations that did not focus on court, but on legal processes prior to court (e.g., interpreters used at police stations, or during the forensic examination) or after court (e.g., during detention).

Table 2.
Eligibility criteria based on the PIO framework for including studies in this scoping review.

All publications identified following the data-based search were exported into the reference management software, Mendeley, and thereafter, screened.

2.4 Chart and weigh the data

The charting and weighting process involved all three authors. The first author used the data extraction tool to extract data from each publication. This included general information about the author, data and source of publication, descriptive information about the participants as well as information pertaining to the accommodations. This tool contained working definitions for all constructs measured and data was captured in an Excel spreadsheet.

For the purpose of this study, a broad classification of disability types that could result in communication disability were used. The groups include intellectual

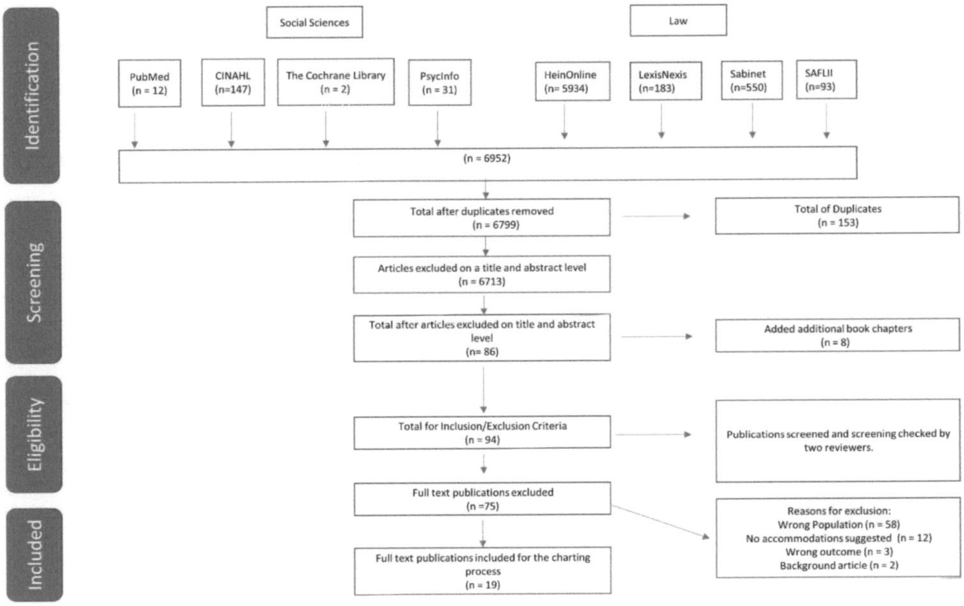

Figure 1.
PRISMA study selection flow diagram.

disability (an impairment in intellectual functions such as reasoning, problem solving and abstract thinking); hearing disability (hearing loss that prevents children relying on auditory input, hence impacting on speech and language development); deaf-blindness disability (a dual sensory impairment); communication disability (an impairment in speech, language and/or communication); physical disability (a permanent and significant limit to the child's physical ability); ASD (a persistent impairment in social communication and social interaction across multiple contexts); and multiple disabilities (any combination of any of the above-mentioned impairments) [47]. This classification has been used only for descriptive purposes. After the extracted data had been entered in the Excel spreadsheet, a high level of inter-rater agreement (97%) was calculated, pointing to very good interrater reliability.

For the purposes of the current study, weighting was based on the frequency with which each accommodation had been reported. Each accommodation was counted in terms of frequency and ranked from highest (i.e., mentioned most frequently) to lowest.

2.5 Conduct the analysis and report the results

An inductive coding approach was used to identify, synthesize and classify themes related to court accommodations [48]. All three authors engaged in this iterative process of reflecting on emerging themes and categories by reviewing publications and coming together to summarize key themes in the data. Points of disagreement were discussed in online team meetings until consensus was reached. Once the court accommodations had been identified, they were classified according to themes [49] in the court accommodation guidelines namely: (i) Children should be allowed to use their preferred 'voice'—irrespective of the communication method or mode—throughout the whole legal process; (ii) Children should be shown respect and treated with dignity by all persons involved throughout the legal process; (iii) Children should feel that all decisions are being made in a fair and neutral way throughout the whole legal process; and (iv) Children should feel that all legal practitioners can be trusted and that their decisions are easy to understand and in the child's best interest.

3. Findings

The findings of this legal scoping review are presented as descriptive information related to the 19 included articles (i.e., authors, year of publication, type of publication, and the country in which the court accommodation was granted) as well as information on the Population (i.e., the type of disability that the children had), the Intervention (i.e., the types of accommodations) and finally the outcomes (i.e., whether accommodations reflect national or international law, the type of court in which the case was heard, as well as any specific laws that were mentioned). **Table 1** includes descriptive information as well as information related to the Population and Outcomes, while **Table 3** contains the bulk of the data and the main emphasis of the research, namely the accommodations.

3.1 Descriptive information on included papers

Descriptive characteristics of included publications (N = 19) are summarized in **Table 1**. Despite the search starting in 2006 (following the adoption of the CRPD), the earliest papers included were from 2012 (3 papers, #2, 10, 18); five from 2014 (including four book chapters from the same international book, #3, 4, 5, 13 as well as a journal paper (#15); one from 2015 (#12); four from 2016 (#1, 6, 11, 16) and three each from 2017 (#8, 9, 14) and 2018 (#7, 17, 19). Despite alerts being put up, no later relevant papers were flagged. It is also interesting to note that by far the majority of papers (12/19 = 63%) were published in international peer-reviewed journals, comprising nine law journals, two multi-disciplinary journals and one social sciences journal. Five book chapters were also included (#3, 4, 5, 11, 13), a research paper (#10) as well as a master's thesis (#16). The majority of studies were concerned with the status quo in the UK and its affiliates, comprising the UK (#7, 11, 13, 17), Ireland (#8, 9, 10, 11, 16, 17); England (#2) and Wales (#9) followed by six studies in South Africa (#2, 4, 6, 11, 18, 19), then four in the USA (#1, 5, 11, 15), three in Australia (#12, 16, 17), two in Israel (#3, 16), and one each in Canada (#2), Malawi (#14) and Bulgaria (#11). Five studies referred to more than one country (#2, 9, 11, 16, 17).

Next an analysis was made of the different types of childhood disability that the accommodations specifically referred to (i.e., addressing the population construct). Just more than half of the studies (10/19 = 52.6%) (#1, 6, 7, 12, 13, 14, 16, 17, 18, 19) did not refer to a specific type of disability while five referred to multiple types of disability (#2, 3, 5, 9, 11) with four referring to only one type of disability (# 4, 8, 10, 15). Regarding the specific type of disability, six papers each focused on intellectual disability (#2, 3, 8, 9, 10, 11), physical disability (#2, 3, 5, 9, 11, 15), five on communication disability (#3, 4, 5, 9, 11) and one each on ASD (#5), multiple disability (#2) and hearing disability (#11).

When unpacking the Outcomes (i.e., whether the laws are national or international, the types of courts represented and the specific laws mentioned), interesting observations were made. An almost equal split was seen between studies mentioning both national and international laws, with nine studies mentioning both (#3, 4, 6, 7, 10, 11, 12, 14, 17) and only one study more mentioning only national laws (#1, 2, 5, 8, 9, 13, 15,16, 18, 19). No studies mentioned only international law—always domesticating the

Accommodations				
#	**Guideline 1** ***Children should be allowed to use their preferred 'voice'***	**Guideline 2** ***Children should be shown respect and treated with dignity***	**Guideline 3** ***Children should feel that all decisions are being made in a fair and neutral way***	**Guideline 4** ***Children should feel that all legal practitioners can be trusted***
1	• Use AAC • Use a sign language interpreter • Allow communication enhancements	• Ensure physical accessibility • Allow support person • Allow support animal • Allow stuffed animal • Modify the courtroom setup	—	• Use modified oath • Allow leading questions
2	• Use an intermediary • Use a sign language interpreter	• Allow support person • Testify behind a screen • Testify via live video/ television link • Testify outside courtroom • Use CCTV in court	• Allow video/ pre-recorded evidence	• Allow judicial officers' intervention
3	• Involve a special investigator • Use AAC • Use AAC toolkit • Use an interpreter	• Conduct trial in camera • Testify behind a screen • Testify outside the courtroom • Allow frequent breaks • Testify not on the witness stand • Testify in the judge's chambers • Testify without the defendant present in the courtroom, and only the defense attorney present	• Remove official attire • Involve an expert professional • Involve an expert witness	• Use facilitator (to simplify language, give meaning and to support) • Allow linguistic simplification
4	• Use an intermediary • Use AAC • Use anatomical dolls • Obtain a victim impact statement	• Testify outside the courtroom • Develop specialized services for persons who use AAC • Conduct a functional assessment of individual	• Involve an expert witness • Film proceedings to review the communication	• Allow linguistic simplification • Use appropriate and proper questioning strategies
5	• Use AAC • Use interpreter • Use sign language interpreter • Use facilitated communication	—	—	• Allow leading questions
6	• Use an intermediary	• Ensure physical accessibility • Use CCTV in court • Conduct informal court proceedings in a relaxed and non-adversarial environment	—	• Use appropriate and proper questioning strategies

Accommodations				
#	**Guideline 1** *Children should be allowed to use their preferred 'voice'*	**Guideline 2** *Children should be shown respect and treated with dignity*	**Guideline 3** *Children should feel that all decisions are being made in a fair and neutral way*	**Guideline 4** *Children should feel that all legal practitioners can be trusted*
7	• Use an intermediary	—	—	• Use appropriate and proper questioning strategies • Disallow tag questions • Disallow leading questions
8	• Use an intermediary	• Testify behind a screen • Testify via live video/ television link	• Remove official attire • Allow video/ pre-recorded evidence • Prohibit personal cross-examination by accused or defendant • Allow sworn depositions	—
9	• Use AAC • Use an intermediary	• Testify via live video/ television link • Allow the functional assessment of individual	• Remove official attire • Allow video/ pre-recorded evidence	• Allow judicial officers' intervention • Use appropriate and proper questioning
10	• Use an intermediary • Use a sign language interpreter • Obtain a victim impact statement • Allow video/ prerecorded evidence • Allow out-of court testimony	• Ensure physical accessibility • Testify via live video/ television link • Use CCTV in court • Make information accessible for those with visual and hearing impairments	• Remove official attire	• Allow judicial officers' intervention • Provide information about the proceedings in plain language, Braille, accessible and child-friendly format
11	• Use AAC • Use a sign language interpreter • Use facilitated communication	• Ensure physical accessibility • Use auxiliary hearing devices • Allow Guardian ad Litem	• Appoint an *Amicus Curiae*	• Provide real-time captioning of court proceedings • Appoint independent advocate
12	• Use AAC • Use an intermediary	• Allow support person • Testify behind a screen • Testify outside courtroom • Conduct trial in camera • Use CCTV in court	• Remove official attire	• Use appropriate and proper questioning strategies • Familiarize witness with and explain the legal process and court procedures

Accommodations				
#	**Guideline 1** ***Children should be allowed to use their preferred 'voice'***	**Guideline 2** ***Children should be shown respect and treated with dignity***	**Guideline 3** ***Children should feel that all decisions are being made in a fair and neutral way***	**Guideline 4** ***Children should feel that all legal practitioners can be trusted***
13	• Use an intermediary	• Testify behind a screen • Testify via live video/ television link • Conduct trial in camera • Allow frequent breaks • Address witness by name to ensure his/her concentration	• Remove official attire • Allow video/ pre-recorded evidence	• Use appropriate and proper questioning strategies • Disallow tag questions
14	• Use AAC • Use a sign language interpreter • Use an intermediary	• Ensure physical accessibility • Provide materials in Braille and other accessible formats • Relook terminology that carries stigma and discrimination • Allow guides to assist with accessibility	—	• Provide readers to assist with access to information
15	• Use AAC • Use an intermediary	• Ensure physical accessibility • Allow stuffed animal • Conduct trial in camera • Use CCTV in court • Allow Guardian ad Litem • Allow enough and extra time for testifying • Allow a familiar person to help the court to interpret and understand a child's needs and disability throughout the process	• Involve expert professional	• Use appropriate and proper questioning strategies • Forbid protracted questioning of children • Forbid continuances that cause needless delay of the trial
16	• Use AAC • Use an intermediary • Give evidence through free narration (no questioning)	• Testify via live/ television link • Allow individualized support	• Remove official attire • Allow video/ pre-recorded evidence	• Use pictures/ communication aids to enhance understanding
17	• Use AAC • Use an intermediary • Give evidence through free narration (no questioning)	• Testify via live/ television link	• Remove official attire • Allow video/ pre-recorded evidence	—
18	• Use an intermediary	• Use CCTV in court	—	—
19	• Use AAC	• Allow support person	• Involve expert witness	• Allow linguistic simplification

Accommodations				
#	**Guideline 1** ***Children should be allowed to use their preferred 'voice'***	**Guideline 2** ***Children should be shown respect and treated with dignity***	**Guideline 3** ***Children should feel that all decisions are being made in a fair and neutral way***	**Guideline 4** ***Children should feel that all legal practitioners can be trusted***
	• Use an intermediary • Use anatomical dolls	• Modify the setup of the courtroom • Conduct trial in camera • Use CCTV in court • Allow frequent breaks • Address the child with a disability by name and wait for him/her to make eye contact		• Use appropriate and proper questioning strategies

Note: AAC = Augmentative and Alternative Communication; CCTV = closed circuit television.

Table 3.
Court accommodations identified in publications (the # in ***Table 3*** *correspond with the # in* ***Table 1****).*

international law (e.g., the CRPD or CRC) with national laws. A variety of courts were mentioned, with the criminal court system being mentioned most frequently in 15 papers (#2, 3, 5, 6, 8, 9, 10, 11, 12, 14, 15, 16, 17, 18, 19). Children's court (presiding over civil and criminal matters) was mentioned once (#6); as was the Supreme Court, and the Court of Appeal (#5), and the South African Equality Court, European Court of Human Rights, and the High Court (#11). Four papers did not mention any particular courts (# 1, 4, 7, 13). **Table 1** also includes a number of specific laws that were cited in the papers, but for the sake of brevity they are not analyzed any further. Thereafter in **Table 3**, a thematic analysis of the interventions that were described in the various papers (i.e., the specific accommodations) was done.

Across the 19 included papers, a total of 165 accommodations were mentioned, of which the majority was related to Guideline 2 (Respect) (65/165), followed by Guideline 1 (Voice) 48/165, Guideline 4 (Trust) (29/165) and finally Guideline 3 (Fairness) (23/165).

Under Guideline 2 (Respect), the use of CCTV (n = 7, 11%) and to be allowed to testify via live/television link (n = 7, 11%) were mentioned the most frequently. Under Guideline 1 (Voice), the use of an intermediary (n = 15, 31%) and the use of Augmentative and Alternative Communication (AAC) (n = 12, 25%) were mentioned the most frequently. Under Guideline 4 (Trust), the use of appropriate and proper questioning strategies (n = 8, 30%) was mentioned the most, and thereafter allowing linguistic simplification (n = 3, 10%) and allowing intervention by judicial officers (n = 3, 10%) were mentioned the most frequently. And lastly, under Guideline 3 (Fairness), removal of official attire (n = 8, 35%) and allowing video/pre-recorded evidence (n = 6, 26%) was mentioned the most frequently.

4. Discussion

This scoping review aimed to identify accommodations that have been afforded to abused children with communication disabilities across the world to enable then to participate in court. Results showed that court accommodations are indeed highlighted by both legal and social science disciplines and furthermore, has been referred to in international and national law. Affording abused children with communication disabilities accommodations to improve the quality of their participation in court will promote child well-being and enhance the integrity of justice for all children [50]. The specific court accommodations identified in this review could ensure effective access to justice for abused children with communication disabilities.

The first guideline focused on ensuring that the child's voice is being heard in court and on the accommodations that could assist children to express themselves in court. The use of intermediaries was the one accommodation highlighted most frequently. Most countries have an intermediary system in place, and research has highlighted the advantages of using intermediaries in court and how they can improve the communication for children [51–54]. The main role of the intermediary is to protect the child from any difficulties experienced in testifying in court and giving evidence, and furthermore, facilitate a friendly court environment for the child with a communication disability [54]. However, it must be noted, that one accommodation alone is typically not effective to ensure effective participation in court for all children, and therefore, a variety of accommodations must be considered and accepted [38, 55]. An additional accommodation that was frequently mentioned under Guideline 1, was the use of AAC. AAC can be defined as a set of tools and strategies (including spoken and written modes of communication) that a child with a communication disability can use to solve daily communicative challenges [56]. Examples of AAC include gestures, sign languages, as well as object and graphic symbols that can be displayed on communication boards or on electronic devices with voice output. It is crucial for courts to be more accommodating and to recognize the diverse communication methods used by children with communication disabilities that could enable them to participate in court (i.e., to testify) [57].

The second guideline focused on the child with a communication disability being shown respect and treated with dignity. The use of closed-circuit television (CCTV) and to allow testimony via live/television link were the two court accommodations mentioned the most frequently under this guideline. A CCTV set-up can be used to protect the child with a communication disability during testimony, giving the people in the courtroom sight of the separate room [36, 58, 59]. Giving evidence via live/television link has also proven to reduce the child's exposure to the harsh and unfriendly courtroom environment [60].

The third guideline focused on the child with a communication disability's feeling that all decisions are being made in a fair and neutral manner. Court accommodations that were mentioned most frequently were removal of official attire and allowing video/pre-recorded evidence. Research has shown that the removal of official attire is also linked to child witnesses feeling more comfortable and at ease in the courtroom, and therefore, assisting the child in giving improved evidence in court [39, 55, 61, 62]. Allowing pre-recorded evidence has also been documented and has been used effectively in countries such as England and Wales [63], and could assist the child witness with a communication disability to provide quality evidence in court [55, 64].

Finally, the fourth guideline focused on how the child with a communication disability could feel that all legal practitioners can be trusted. Court accommodations mentioned were the use of appropriate and proper questioning strategies, allowing linguistic simplification and allowing judicial officers intervention. Children with communication disabilities are less likely to understand the legal language used by legal practitioners [50, 64]. The complexity of legal language creates knowledge and information gaps, causes isolation of the child witness and decreases trust in the legal system as an equal and fair system [65]. Allowing the use of appropriate questioning strategies and linguistic simplification (which is the process of editing and processing written and spoken information to ensure that it is simple, clear and easy to understand) could benefit the child witness in understanding important legal information about the court procedures as well as the questions asked in court [66].

5. Limitations

One limitation of this review is its inclusion of only English-language material. It is also possible that not all relevant publications were identified, as gray literature or reports pertaining to experiences of children with disabilities in the criminal justice system were excluded.

6. Conclusion

This legal scoping review sought to identify the specific court accommodations that have been reported in literature and that could enable abused children with communication disabilities to participate in court. Different court accommodations were identified and focused on the four court accommodation guidelines developed by White [49] that centered around voice, respect, fairness and trust. Abuse of children with communication disabilities, including sexual abuse, is a grave and devasting problem in society. The legal scholar, Keane [67] stated that while there may not be any official figures for the number of children with communication disabilities appearing as sexually abused witnesses in criminal cases, it appears as if the numbers are escalating within this group. Therefore, it is of utmost importance that court accommodations for children with communication disabilities is recognized and made available to support and enable their participation in court as witnesses. Every effort should be made to support abused children with communication disabilities in their pursuit of access to justice, but more importantly, in their pursuit of their basic rights as children.

Acknowledgements

The librarians, specifically at the Law and Humanities Faculty at the University of Pretoria are gratefully acknowledged for their assistance and knowledgeable input into the review process. The authors would also like to acknowledge that the data included in this publication formed part of the doctorate thesis titled, "Accommodating persons with severe communication disabilities in court: Development and appraisal of guidelines" by Robyn White at the University of Pretoria, South Africa prepared under the supervision of the first and third authors. This PhD study was funded by the National Institute for the Humanities and Social Sciences (NIHSS) in collaboration with the South African Humanities Deans Association (SAHUDA) and the second author would like to acknowledge her financial contributors and their financial assistance towards this research. Opinions expressed and conclusions arrived at are those of the authors and cannot necessarily be attributed to the NIHSS and SAHUDA.

Authors' contributions

J.B, R.W. and E.J. contributed to the study conceptualization, methodology development, data analysis, critical analysis and review, visualizing the work. J.B. and R.W. contributed to writing the original draft and revision.

Author details

Juan Bornman, Robyn White* and Ensa Johnson
University of Pretoria, South Africa

*Address all correspondence to: robynwilson13@gmail.com

References

[1] World Health Organization. INSPIRE: Seven Strategies for Ending Violence against Children. Geneva, Switzerland: WHO; 2016

[2] Hillis S, Mercy J, Amobi A, Kress H. Global prevalence of past-year violence against children: A systematic review and minimum estimates. Pediatrics. 2016; **137**(3)

[3] Maguire-Jack K, Font SA. Community and individual risk factors for physical child abuse and child neglect: Variations by poverty status. Child Maltreatment. 2017;**22**(3):215-226

[4] Araten-Bergman T, Bigby C, Ritchie G. Literature review of best practice supports in disability services for the prevention of abuse of people with disability. Reports in Disability Service Commission. 2017:1-45. Available from: https://www.researchgate.net/publication/341448390_Literature_Review_of_Best_Practice_Supports_in_Disability_Services_for_the_Prevention_of_Abuse_of_People_with_Disability

[5] Doidge JC, Higgins DJ, Delfabbro P, Segal L. Risk factors for child maltreatment in an Australian population-based birth cohort. Child Abuse & Neglect. 2017;**64**:47-60

[6] Flynn S. Theorizing disability in child protection: Applying critical disability studies to the elevated risk of abuse for disabled children. Disabil Society. 2020; **35**(6):949-971

[7] Svensson B, Eriksson UB, Janson S. Exploring risk for abuse of children with chronic conditions or disabilities—Parent's perceptions of stressors and the role of professionals. Child: Care, Health and Development. 2013;**39**(6): 887-893

[8] Murphy N. Maltreatment of children with disabilities: The breaking point. Journal of Child Neurology. 2011;**26**(8): 1054-1056

[9] Algood CL, Hong JS, Gourdine RM, Williams AB. Maltreatment of children with developmental disabilities: An ecological systems analysis. Children and Youth Services Review. 2011;**33**(7): 1142-1148

[10] Briggs F. Child sexual abuse in early-childhood care and education settings. Early Child Development and Care. 2014;**184**(9–10):1415-1435

[11] Sullivan J, Beech A. Professional perpetrators: Sex offenders who use their employment to target and sexually abuse the children with whom they work. Child Abuse Review Journal of British Association Study Prevent Child Abuse Neglect. 2002;**11**(3):153-167

[12] Devries K, Kuper H, Knight L, Allen E, Kyegombe N, Banks LM, et al. Reducing physical violence toward primary school students with disabilities. Journal of Adolescent Health. 2017;**62**: 303-310

[13] Namy S, Carlson C, Norcini Pala A, Faris D, Knight L, Allen E, et al. Gender, violence and resilience among Ugandan adolescents. Child Abuse & Neglect. 2017;**70**:303-314

[14] Zeanah CH, Humphreys KL. Child abuse and neglect. Journal of the American Academy of Child and Adolescent Psychiatry. 2018;**57**(9):637-644

[15] Brown J, Cohen P, Johnson JG, Salzinger S. A longitudinal analysis of risk factors for child maltreatment: Findings of a 17-year prospective study of officially recorded and self-reported

child abuse and neglect. Child Abuse & Neglect. 1998;**22**(11):1065-1078

[16] Dion J, Paquette G, Tremblay K-N, Collin-Vézina D, Chabot M. Child maltreatment among children with intellectual disability in the Canadian incidence study. American Journal on Intellectual and Developmental Disabilities. 2018;**123**(2):176-192

[17] McDonnell CG, Boan AD, Bradley CC, Seay KD, Charles JM, Carpenter LA. Child maltreatment in autism spectrum disorder and intellectual disability: Results from a population-based sample. Journal of Child Psychology and Psychiatry. 2019; **60**(5):576-584

[18] Bornman J. Preventing abuse and providing access to justice for individuals with complex communication needs: The role of augmentative and alternative communication. Seminars in Speech and Language. 2017;**38**(4):321-331

[19] Hellström L. A systematic review of polyvictimization among children with attention deficit hyperactivity or autism spectrum disorder. International Journal of Environmental Research and Public Health. 2019;**16**(13):2280

[20] Helton JJ, Lightfoot E, Fu QJ, Bruhn CM. Prevalence and severity of child impairment in a US sample of child maltreatment investigations. Journal of Developmental and Behavioral Pediatrics. 2019;**40**(4):285-292

[21] Jones L, Bellis MA, Wood S, Hughes K, McCoy E, Eckley L, et al. Prevalence and risk of violence against children with disabilities: A systematic review and meta-analysis of observational studies. Lancet. 2012; **380**(9845):899-907

[22] Westcott HL, Jones DPH. Annotation: The abuse of disabled children. The Journal of Child Psychology and Psychiatry and Allied Disciplines. 1999;**40**(4):497-506

[23] Sobsey D, Doe T. Patterns of sexual abuse and assault. Sexuality and Disability. 1991;**9**(3):243-259

[24] Nyberg A, Ferm U, Bornman J. School-based abuse prevention programs for children with disabilities: A qualitative study of components and methods. Australas J Spec Incl Educ [Internet]. 2021;**45**(2):252-267

[25] Barron I, Allardyce S, Young H, Levit R. Exploration of the relationship between severe and complex disabilities and child sexual abuse: A call for relevant research. Journal of Child Sexual Abuse. 2019;**28**(7):759-780

[26] Ford JD, Delker BC. Polyvictimization in childhood and its adverse impacts across the lifespan: Introduction to the special issue. Journal of Trauma Dissociation [Internet]. 2018; **19**(3):275-288

[27] MacIntosh J, Wuest J, Ford-Gilboe M, Varcoe C. Cumulative effects of multiple forms of violence and abuse on women. Violence Vict [Internet]. 2015; **30**(3):502-521

[28] Harrell E. Crime Against Persons with Disabilities, 2009–2012—Statistical Tables [Internet]. 2012. Available from: https://bjs.ojp.gov/library/publications/crime-against-persons-disabilities-2009-2012-statistical-tables

[29] Åker TH, Johnson MS. Sexual abuse and violence against people with intellectual disability and physical impairments: Characteristics of police-investigated cases in a Norwegian national sample. Journal of Applied

Research in Intellectual Disabilities. 2020;**33**:139-145

[30] Nareadi PT. Influences on under reporting of sexual abuse of teenagers with intellectual disability: Results and implications of a South African Study. Journal of Psychology in Africa. 2013 Jan;**23**(4):625-629

[31] Covington T. The public health approach for understanding and preventing child maltreatment: A brief review of the literature and a call to action. Child Welfare. 2013;**92**(2): 21-39

[32] O'Donnell M, Scott D, Stanley F. Child abuse and neglect—Is it time for a public health approach? Australian and New Zealand Journal of Public Health. 2008;**32**(4):325-330

[33] Bryen DN, Wickman C. Testifying in court in the USA. In: Bryen DN, Bornman J, editors. Stop Violence against People with Disabilities! An International Resource. Pretoria: Pretoria University Law Press; 2014. pp. 161-178

[34] White R, Bornman J, Johnson E. Testifying in court as a victim of crime for persons with little or no functional speech: Vocabulary implications. Child Abus Res A South African J [Internet]. 2015;**16**(1):1-14

[35] Edwards C, Harold G, Kilcommins S. Access to Justice for People with Disabilities as Victims of Crime in Ireland [Internet]. 2012. Available from: https://cora.ucc.ie/bitstream/handle/10468/6966/Access_to_Justice_for_People_with_Disabilities_as_Victims_of_Crime_in_Ireland_2012.pdf?sequence=1&isAllowed=y

[36] Fambasayi R. The right to protection of children testifying in criminal proceedings. South Africa: North-West University; 2016. pp. 1-59. Available from: http://repository.nwu.ac.za/handle/10394/25347 [mini-dissertation]

[37] Bhojani SH, Bhatt N. Data mining techniques and trends—A review. Global Journal of Research Analysis. 2018; **August**:1-4

[38] White R, Bornman J, Johnson E, Msipa D. Court accommodations for persons with severe communication disabilities: A legal scoping review. Psychology, Public Policy, and Law. 2021;**27**(3):399-420

[39] Beckene T, Forrester-Jones R, Murphy GH. Experiences of going to court: Witnesses with intellectual disabilities and their carers speak up. J Appl Res Intellect Disabil [Internet]. 2017:1-12

[40] Arksey H and, O'Malley L. Scoping studies: Towards a methodological framework. International Journal of Social Research Methodology 2005;8(1): 19–32

[41] The Joanna Briggs Institute. The Joanna Briggs Institute Reviewers' Manual 2015: Methodology for JBI scoping reviews [Internet]. 2015. Available from: https://nursing.lsuhsc.edu/JBI/docs/ReviewersManuals/Scoping-.pdf

[42] Baude W, Chilton AS, Malani A. Making doctrinal work more rigorous: Lessons from systematic reviews. Univ Chicago Law Rev [Internet]. 2017;**84**(1): 37-58

[43] Aslam S, Emmanuel P. Formulating a researchable question: A critical step for facilitating good clinical research. Indian Journal of Sexual Transmission Diseases. 2010;**31**(1):47-50

[44] United Nations. The Convention on the Rights of the Child [Internet]. 1989.

Available from: https://www.unicef.org/child-rights-convention/convention-text

[45] The American Psychiatric Association. What is mental illness? [Internet]. 2020. Available from: https://www.psychiatry.org/patients-families/what-is-mental-illness

[46] Moher D, Liberati A, Tetzlaff J, Altman DG, The PRISMA Group. Preferred reporting items for systematic reviews and meta-analyses: The PRISMA statement. PLoS Medicine. 2009;**6**(7)

[47] Bianquin N, Bulgarelli D. Conceptual review of disabilities. In: Besio S, Bulgarelli D, Stancheva-Popkostadinova V, editors. Play Development in Children with Disabilties [Internet]. Berlin/Boston: Walter de Gruyter GmbH & Co KG; 2016. pp. 1-228

[48] Fereday J, Muir-Cochrane E. Demonstrating rigor using thematic analysis: A hybrid approach of inductive and deductive coding and theme development. International Journal of Qualitative Methods [Internet]. 2006; **5**(1):80-92

[49] White RM. Accommodating Persons with Severe Communication Disabilities in Court: Development and Appraisal of Guidelines. Pretoria: University of Pretoria; 2021

[50] Murphy W. Traumatized children who participate in legal proceedings are entitled to testimonial and participatory accommodations under the americans with disabilities act. Roger Williams University Law Review [Internet]. 2014; **19**:361-381

[51] Plotnikoff J, Woolfson R. Intermediaries in the Criminal Justice System. Bristol: Policy Press; 2015. pp. 1-338

[52] Matthias CR, Zaal FN. Intermediaries for child witnesses: Old problems, new solutions and judicial differences in South Africa. International Journal of Child Rights [Internet]. 2011; **19**(2):251-269

[53] Jonker G, Swanzen R. Intermediary services for child witnesses testyfying in the South African Criminal Courts. International Journal of Human Rights [Internet]. 2007;**6**:90-113

[54] Fambasayi R, Koraan R. Intermediaries and the international obligation to protect child witnesses in South Africa. Potchefstroom Electron Law Journal. 2018;**21**(21):1-30

[55] Doak J, Doak L. Non-verbal victims in the adversarial criminal process: Communication, competency, and credibility. Northern Ireland Legal Quarterly. 2017;**68**:451-468

[56] Beukelman DR, Light JC. Augmentative and Alternative Communication: Supporting Children and Adults with Complex Communication Needs. Fifth ed. Baltimore, MD: Paul H. Brookes Publishing; 2020. pp. 1-686

[57] Flynn E. Disabled Justice? Access to Justice and the UN Convention on the Rights of Persons with Disabilities. New York: Routledge/Taylor & Francis Group; 2016

[58] Matthias C. Protecting child witnesses: New developments and implications for social workers. Social Work. 2011;**47**(2):195-204

[59] Carter E, Boezaart T. Article 13 of the United Nations convention on the rights of people with disabilities: Does

the Children 's Act 38 of 2005 support access to justice for children with disabilities ? Journal of Contempt Roman Law. 2016;**79**:248-260

[60] O'Leary C, Feely M. Alignment of the Irish legal system and Article 13.1 of the CRPD for witnesses with communication difficulties. Disability Studies Quarterly. 2018;**38**(1):1-22

[61] O'Leary C. Accommodations for witnesses with communication difficulties in Irish criminal proceedings: An examination in relation to Article 13.1 [Internet]. 2016. Available from: http://ir.obihiro.ac.jp/dspace/handle/10322/3933

[62] Equality and Human Rights Commission. Inclusive justice: A system designed for all [Internet]. 2020. Available from: https://www.equalityhumanrights.com/sites/default/files/ehrc_inclusive_justice_a_system_designed_for_all_june_2020.pdf

[63] Beqiraj J, Mcnamara L, Wicks V. Access to Justice for Persons with Disabilities: From International Principles to Practice. International Bar Association; 2017. Available from: https://binghamcentre.biicl.org/projects/access-to-justice-for-persons-with-disabilities-from-international-principles-to-practice

[64] Morrison J, Forrester-Jones R, Bradshaw J, Murphy G. Communication and cross-examination in court for children and adults with intellectual disabilities: A systematic review. International Journal of Evidence Proof. 2019;**23**(4):366-398

[65] Mor S. With access and justice for all. Cardozo Law Review. 2017;**39**:611

[66] BenZeev N, Lerner N, Klein Y. The right of people with disabilities to legal justice: A view from Israel. In: Bryen DN, Bornman J, editors. Stop Violence against People with Disabilities! An International Resource. Pretoria: Pretoria University Law Press; 2014. pp. 105-135

[67] Keane A. Cross-examination of vulnerable witnesses—Towards a blueprint for re-professionalisation. International Journal of Evidence Proof. 2012;**16**(2):175-198